Anti-Inflammatory Drinks

Drinks
for Health

**100 Smoothies, Shots, Teas,
Broths, and Seltzers to Help**
Prevent Disease • Lose Weight • Increase Energy
Look Radiant • Reduce Pain • *and More!*

MARYEA FLAHERTY
Founder of HappyHealthyMama.com

Adams Media
New York London Toronto Sydney New Delhi

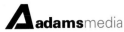

Adams Media
An Imprint of Simon & Schuster, Inc.
57 Littlefield Street
Avon, Massachusetts 02322

First Adams Media trade paperback edition February 2019

ADAMS MEDIA and colophon are trademarks of Simon & Schuster.

For information about special discounts for bulk purchases, please contact Simon & Schuster Special Sales at 1-866-506-1949 or business@simonandschuster.com.

The Simon & Schuster Speakers Bureau can bring authors to your live event. For more information or to book an event contact the Simon & Schuster Speakers Bureau at 1-866-248-3049 or visit our website at www.simonspeakers.com.

Interior design by Heather McKiel
Photographs by James Stefiuk
Nutritional statistics by Melinda Boyd

Manufactured in the United States of America

10 9 8 7 6 5 4 3

Library of Congress Cataloging-in-Publication Data has been applied for.

ISBN 978-1-5072-0958-5
ISBN 978-1-5072-0959-2 (ebook)

Contains material adapted from the following title published by Adams Media, an Imprint of Simon & Schuster, Inc.: *The Everything® Anti-Inflammation Diet Book* by Karlyn Grimes, MS, RD, LDN, copyright © 2011, ISBN 978-1-4405-1029-8.

Contents

Introduction

From Blueberry Ginger Smoothies and Healthy Hydration Tonics to Mexican Hot Chocolates and Iced Mocha Lattes—fighting inflammation has never been easier or tastier. Filled with delicious recipes for smoothies, juices, teas, tonics, and more, *Anti-Inflammatory Drinks for Health* is packed with one hundred healthful drinks that will help you battle against chronic inflammation and its harmful consequences.

What is inflammation? Inflammation is your body's normal response to injury or attack by bacteria, pathogens, or irritants. It's your immune system's natural and necessary function when it needs to fight against something potentially harmful. However, when your inflammation response does not stop working and continues to function long after the original need, the results can be damaging.

This constant state of inflammation, called *chronic inflammation*, can be caused by certain lifestyle choices. Excess weight and activities such as ongoing stress and lack of sleep are all factors that can keep your body in a pro-inflammatory state on an ongoing basis. Poor dietary choices and the modern diet of refined carbohydrates, sugar, and overly processed and fried foods also promote chronic inflammation. When your body is in a constant state of inflammation, you are also susceptible to a number of diseases, including cancer, heart disease, Alzheimer's disease, and Parkinson's.

Fortunately, *Anti-Inflammatory Drinks for Health* will help you protect your body from inflammation's harmful effects. This book is designed to help you cut out pro-inflammatory drinks you may already be consuming regularly and replace them with anti-inflammatory, health-promoting drinks. If you can fill your diet with the ingredients in this book, which are all carefully chosen for their anti-inflammatory properties, you will be helping your body win the battle against chronic inflammation.

With this book, you can create delicious and nutritious elixirs that combine the benefits of a wide variety of nutrients and antioxidants to battle inflammation and improve almost every area of life. So, if you're ready to start your journey to less inflammation and better health, then turn the page and let's go!

Chapter 1

UNDERSTANDING INFLAMMATION

Throughout your life, your body is bombarded by toxins, chemicals, viruses, bacteria, and other potentially damaging factors. Fortunately, your body naturally responds to these adverse circumstances by initiating an inflammatory response. During this response, the potentially harmful threats are dealt with promptly and completely. But sometimes that response does not turn off, and you are left with chronic inflammation in your body. A silent enemy, inflammation damages your body and can lead to several debilitating diseases. This chapter will discuss inflammation and some changes you can make to keep it at bay.

What Is Inflammation?

The inflammatory response is completely normal and is the cornerstone of the body's healing response. It is simply the way the body supplies nourishment and enhanced immune activity to areas experiencing injury or infection.

Whenever you are exposed to an infectious agent or experience tissue injury or damage, your immune system mounts an inflammatory response. For example, when you cut your finger and it becomes red and swollen, inflammation goes to work, and it's a lifesaver. Blood flow increases to places that require healing. Pain intensifies as a signal that something is wrong within the body. And compounds such as eicosanoids (also known as *prostaglandins, prostacyclins, thromboxanes,* and *leukotrienes*) are released to attack unwelcome foreign invaders such as bacteria while tending to harmed tissue. Under normal circumstances, once the threat is under control, anti-inflammatory substances are released to turn off the immune response.

The Effects of Chronic Inflammation on the Body

Sometimes, however, inflammation gets the upper hand and continues to operate chronically. This causes continual secretion of pro-inflammatory chemicals in the body. The chronic release and circulation of these chemicals results in an attack on healthy cells, blood vessels, and tissues.

Chronic inflammation generates a wide range of symptoms, including:

- Frequent body aches and pains
- Intermittent infections
- Chronic stiffness
- Loss of joint function
- Recurrent swelling
- Continual congestion
- Persistent indigestion
- Regular bouts of diarrhea
- Unrelenting skin outbreaks

Over time, chronic inflammation acts like a slow but deadly poison, causing overzealous inflammatory chemicals to damage your body as you innocently go about your normal daily activities. The negative consequences associated with out-of-control pro-inflammatory chemicals do not end here. Other diseases and conditions thought to be associated with chronic inflammation include, but are not limited to:

- Allergies
- Anemia
- Asthma
- Cancer
- Crohn's disease
- Congestive heart failure
- Fibromyalgia
- Inflammatory bowel disease (IBD)
- Heart disease
- Kidney failure
- Lupus
- Obesity
- Pancreatitis
- Psoriasis
- Rheumatoid arthritis (RA)
- Stroke

Foods That Increase Inflammation

Research shows that one of the main culprits contributing to chronic inflammation is the food you eat. Certain foods have the ability to trigger inflammation in the body, and when you eat those foods daily, it causes chronic inflammation. It's just as important to stay away from inflammatory foods as it is to add anti-inflammatory foods to your diet. The first step is knowing which foods cause inflammation so you can avoid them!

Advanced Glycation End Products (AGEs)

Researchers have identified chemical reactions that occur in the body that lead to the production of pro-inflammatory substances called *advanced glycation end products* (AGEs). AGEs do not exist in nature but are produced during food processing. Regardless of their source, all AGEs have been shown to exacerbate inflammation.

In a nutshell, the foods high in AGEs are highly processed, refined foods such as:

- Frankfurters, bacon, and powdered egg whites
- Fast foods such as French fries, hamburgers, and fried chicken
- Prepackaged foods that have been preserved, pasteurized, homogenized, or refined, such as white flour, cake mixes, processed cereals, dried milk, dried eggs, pasteurized milk, and canned or frozen precooked meals

- Cream cheese, butter, margarine, and mayonnaise

AGE production is most significant when a mixture of carbohydrates, fats, and proteins is exposed to prolonged thermal processing such as heating, sterilizing, or microwaving. Therefore, foods that have been fried, barbecued, broiled, or cooked in the microwave are more susceptible to higher levels of AGEs.

Trans Fats

Nothing could be more inflammation-promoting than trans fats. These fats lead to the synthesis of pro-inflammatory prostaglandins. Studies have linked high trans fat consumption with high blood levels of CRP (C-reactive protein), the protein linked to inflammation in the body. Foods that tend to be high in trans fats include:

- Fried and deep-fried foods (these are usually cooked in hydrogenated shortening)
- Margarine
- Nondairy creamers
- Shortening
- Baked goods such as cakes, pie crusts, and cookies (especially those with frosting)
- Biscuits
- Frozen breakfast sandwiches
- Doughnuts
- Crackers, chips, and other snack foods that contain the word *hydrogenated* in the ingredient list
- Microwave popcorn

Saturated Fats

Saturated fats are nonessential fats commonly found in meats, high-fat dairy products, and eggs. Although these foods provide important vitamins and minerals, saturated fats can promote inflammation, which is demonstrated by their ability to increase the fibrinogen and CRP inflammatory biomarkers in the blood.

Omega-6 Fatty Acids

Omega-6 fatty acids are a member of the polyunsaturated-fat family. Although they are unsaturated and considered essential in small quantities, excessive intake of omega-6 fatty acids promotes inflammation, encourages blood clotting, and can cause cells in the body to proliferate uncontrollably. The modern diet is weighed down by omega-6 fatty acids because of overconsumption of meats and vegetable oils such as corn, safflower, soybean, and cottonseed that are commonly found in processed foods and fast foods.

Nightshades

Although fruits and vegetables are extremely beneficial to your health, there are certain vegetables that are members of the nightshade family of plants that many claim exacerbate inflammation. These fruits and vegetables include:

- Potatoes
- Tomatoes
- Eggplants
- Sweet and hot peppers (including paprika, cayenne pepper, and Tabasco sauce)
- Ground cherries
- Tomatillos
- Pepinos
- Pimientos

These plants contain a chemical called *solanine*. Anecdotal evidence suggests that solanine may trigger pain and inflammation in some people, but currently there is no research to support the negative claims linked to nightshade vegetables. Individuals with inflammatory conditions can experiment with limiting nightshade vegetables to see if they get any relief from pain and inflammation.

Foods That Fight Inflammation

Now that you know exactly which inflammation-triggering foods you should avoid, what about the good foods? Are there foods that can help control inflammation? Thankfully, there are a myriad of foods that can help your body fight inflammation. In fact, the most powerful inflammation fighters can be found in the grocery store, not the pharmacy! Your best bet is to shop mostly the perimeter of the supermarket where you find fresh, unprocessed foods. Look for a wide variety of brightly colored fruits and vegetables, herbs and spices, and foods with healthy fats. Let's take a closer look at all the inflammation-fighting foods you should be filling your grocery cart up with!

Fruits and Vegetables

Fruits and vegetables are major storehouses of phytochemicals and antioxidants, both of which have anti-inflammatory powers. Phytochemicals are chemicals found in plants, and although they are not essential for life, their benefits are far-reaching, such as helping to reduce the risk of cancer, heart disease, and diabetes. Plants rely on phytochemicals for their own protection and survival. These potent chemicals help plants resist the attacks of bacteria and fungi, the potential havoc brought on by free radicals, and the constant exposure to ultraviolet light from the sun. Fortunately, when we consume plants, the plants' chemicals infuse into our body's tissues and provide ammunition against disease.

In a similar manner to phytochemicals, antioxidants halt and repair free radical damage throughout the body. The most potent antioxidants include vitamin A, vitamin C, vitamin E, and selenium. In addition to fruits and vegetables, these free radical squelchers inhabit whole grains, vegetable oils, nuts, and seeds.

To get the most bang for your buck in the produce section of your local grocery store, choose brightly colored fruits and veggies such as strawberries; blueberries; cantaloupes; spinach; and red, green, and yellow bell peppers. Aim to eat fruits and vegetables that represent each color of the rainbow. It's pretty simple: the more color, the more health benefits. When it comes to fruits, variety is important to ensure you are receiving all the beneficial phytochemicals, antioxidants, vitamins, and minerals while minimizing exposure to any single type of pesticide.

Omega-3 Fatty Acids

Omega-3 fatty acids—polyunsaturated relatives of the omega-6 fatty acid family—have an anti-inflammatory effect in the body. These fatty acids are converted into hormone-like substances called *eicosanoids*. The two most potent omega-3 eicosanoids are eicosapentaenoic acid (EPA) and docosahexaenoic acid (DHA). EPA and DHA have the overall effect of dilating blood vessels, minimizing blood clotting, and reducing inflammation.

Foods high in omega-3s include:

- Fatty fish such as albacore tuna, anchovy, Atlantic herring, halibut, lake trout, mackerel, sardine, stripped sea bass, and wild salmon
- Flaxseeds and flaxseed oils
- Walnuts
- Soybeans
- Tofu

Probiotics

All humans have millions and millions of naturally occurring bacteria in their bodies. Normally, bacteria get a bad rap, but the right types of bacteria, specifically lactobacilli and bifidobacteria, can keep you healthy and even prevent disease. More specifically, these bacteria support the immune system, keeping it strong and better able to fend off disease and illness. They also have anti-inflammatory effects in the gut that can be helpful in treating constipation, diarrhea, inflammatory bowel disease, and irritable bowel syndrome.

You can help good bacteria flourish by consuming foods that contain high concentrations of healthy probiotics (the term *probiotics* means "for life") such as Lactobacillus acidophilus. Fermented milk products such as yogurt, kefir, and some soy-based beverages will increase the probiotic bacteria within your body. Look on the label for the "live and active cultures" statement to ensure that you are increasing your consumption of probiotics.

Lean Protein

Dietary protein is responsible for the growth, maintenance, and repair of the body, but can also contribute to chronic disease development if not chosen properly and in the correct amounts. Lean meats; white-meat poultry; and eggs, on the other hand, will give you clean protein without excessive amounts of pro-inflammatory fats. Cold-water fish offer plenty of quality protein with a kick of anti-inflammatory omega-3 fatty acids.

Vegetable proteins, such as soy foods, beans, lentils, whole grains, seeds, and nuts, will further reduce the presence of pro-inflammatory agents in the body while giving you a blast of phytochemicals and antioxidants.

Garlic

Garlic is a potent anti-inflammatory power food. It contains chemicals that crush the inflammation-promoting substances in the body. As a result, regular garlic consumption can help minimize the side effects of asthma and reduce the pain and inflammation associated with osteoarthritis and rheumatoid arthritis. Garlic can even reduce the production of cancer-causing chemicals that can result when protein is subject to high temperatures through various cooking methods such as grilling.

Curcumin

Curcumin is a substance found in the yellow curry spice turmeric. Curcumin is touted as having antioxidant powers, anti-inflammatory qualities, and possibly even anticancer effects. This spice is popular in India, and some researchers believe there is a link between higher curcumin intake and a lower incidence of Alzheimer's disease. Preliminary findings from animal studies suggest that curcumin may actually possess anti-inflammatory and anti-cancer properties, but currently very little research exists that evaluates the actual effects of curcumin supplementation on disease risk in humans.

Ginger

Ginger is a tropical plant and a relative of turmeric. Certain constituents of ginger, referred to as *gingerols*, are touted to inhibit numerous biochemicals that promote inflammation, especially in cases of osteoarthritis and rheumatoid arthritis. Again, these claims are unsubstantiated, but one thing that ginger has been found to help with is pregnancy-induced nausea and vomiting. Fresh ginger adds a light spiciness and mellow sweetness to dishes and is a wonderful spice to incorporate into stir-fries and dipping sauces.

Lifestyle Choices That Combat and Reduce Inflammation

There are a number of other simple dietary and lifestyle interventions that can keep inflammation from establishing a foothold over the body. Beating inflammation is not just about changing your diet. Your best defensive mode is to combine dietary and lifestyle interventions to ensure that your body is protected.

- **Stay properly hydrated:** Women should aim for 90 ounces of fluids daily, and men should get 125 ounces.
- **Get enough sleep:** Aim for at least seven to nine hours per night.
- **Exercise regularly:** Exercise at least five days per week, including the three essential components of an exercise program: cardiovascular, strengthening, and flexibility.
- **Manage stress:** Take time for yourself every day to chill out and smell the roses. Schedule regular breathing breaks. Research has shown that taking just one large, deep breath can help alleviate stress and its negative effects on the body.
- **Try supplements:** Supplement your diet every day with 1,000 IUs of vitamin D_3 and 1,000 mg of DHA and EPA from fish oils. Be sure to check with your physician before you begin taking a fish oil supplement, especially if you are currently taking any medications.

Chapter 2
SMOOTHIES

Smoothies bring a big nutritional advantage to the table. When you blend whole foods, you get all of the nutrients, from the fiber to the vitamins and minerals. Nothing gets left out! Aptly named, smoothies are smooth, sometimes creamy, and quick and simple to prepare.

Smoothies are the easiest, most versatile way to add anti-inflammatory nutrients to your day. Whether they replace a meal or become your go-to snack, smoothies take minimal effort to blend and are one of the most delicious ways to incorporate a wide variety of anti-inflammatory foods into your diet.

You can, of course, drink a smoothie at any time during the day, but smoothies are especially popular for breakfast. If you have busy mornings, you can prepare all of the ingredients the night before. Then all you have to do in the morning is blend and go!

Since sugar can be inflammatory, I like to keep my smoothies naturally sweetened with fruit. Sometimes I'll add stevia, a natural sweetener made from the stevia plant, if I need to enhance the sweetness a little more. Enjoy the natural sweetness nature provides in these smoothie recipes!

THE PURPLE MACHINE SMOOTHIE

Serves 1

INGREDIENTS

3 large red kale leaves
1 cup unsweetened almond milk
1 cup frozen blueberries
½ medium banana
¼ teaspoon pure stevia powder

1 Tear the kale leaves away from the tough vein in the center. Discard the vein and place the leaves in a large blender with the almond milk.

2 Blend kale leaves and almond milk on high until the kale is completely broken down.

3 Add frozen blueberries, banana, and stevia and blend on high until thoroughly combined and smooth.

4 Consume immediately.

KEY INGREDIENT: Red Kale

Red kale (as well as the blueberries) gives this smoothie a deep purple color, and both are powerful anti-inflammatory agents. Typically, the more color a food has, the more anti-oxidants it contains. The deep color of the kale and blue-berries comes from the antioxidants present in these potent foods. Kale is high in vitamin C and beta-carotene, and these antioxidant vitamins are known to fight damage caused by free radicals. Oxidative stress can lead to inflammation, so those nutrients are helping keep inflammation at bay. Kale has a number of different flavonoids in its leaves, which also come into play in fighting inflammation. In addition, kale is a good source of omega-3 fatty acids and has an ideal ratio of omega-3 fatty acids to omega-6 fatty acids, which is import-ant for fighting inflammation. Omega-3 fatty acids have also been shown to inhibit key inflammatory pathways.

When paired with blueberries, banana, and pure stevia powder, the natural bitter flavor of kale is masked, making this anti-inflammatory smoothie an easy way to get more of the powerhouse leafy green into your diet.

Per Serving
Calories: 184 | Fat: 4.0 g | Protein: 4.4 g | Sodium: 199 mg
Fiber: 8.5 g | Carbohydrates: 38.5 g | Sugar: 21.8 g

STRAWBERRY BEET SMOOTHIE

Serves 1

INGREDIENTS

1 cup whole strawberries, frozen or fresh

1 small beet, peeled and cut into chunks

1 medium banana, peeled and frozen

3 tablespoons chia seeds

2 pitted dates

¼ cup old-fashioned oats

1 cup cold water

1 cup ice

Stevia, to taste (optional)

1 Place all ingredients except stevia in a large blender.

2 Blend the ingredients on high until thoroughly combined and smooth.

3 Taste your smoothie and add stevia if desired.

4 Consume immediately or store in an airtight container in the refrigerator up to 24 hours.

KEY INGREDIENT: Strawberries

This is a vibrant smoothie with a deep pink hue. Deeply pigmented fruits and vegetables are typically high in anti-oxidants, and indeed, strawberries are an excellent source of antioxidant phytochemicals. The antioxidants in strawberries help rid the body of free radicals that promote inflammation. Eating strawberries every week has been shown to lower levels of C-reactive protein, an inflammation marker that is associated with chronic inflammation. Strawberries have also been associated with reducing pain in arthritis patients.

Don't be scared off by the beet in this smoothie. When paired with sweet strawberries and the banana, the beet is mellow and delicious.

Per Serving
Calories: 535 | Fat: 12.1 g | Protein: 15.8 g | Sodium: 69 mg
Fiber: 24.7 g | Carbohydrates: 97.2 g | Sugar: 37.1 g

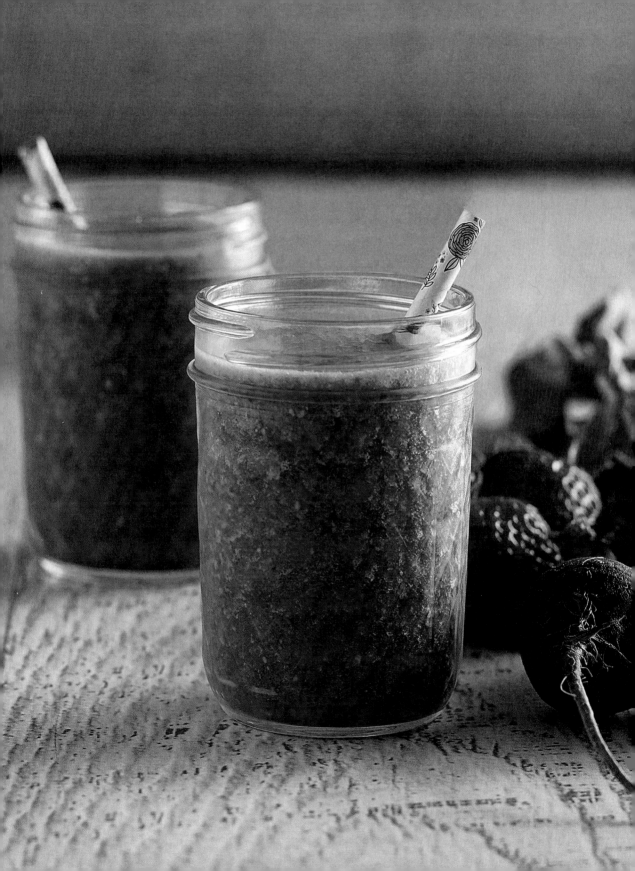

WILD BLUEBERRY POWER SMOOTHIE

Serves 2

INGREDIENTS

1 cup frozen wild blueberries
1 medium banana
1 tablespoon ground flaxseed meal
½ cup chopped parsley
1½ tablespoons peeled, chopped
   ginger
1 cup cold water
2 tablespoons almond butter

---

1 Place all ingredients in a large
   blender.

2 Blend the ingredients on high
   until thoroughly combined and
   smooth.

3 Consume immediately or store
   in an airtight container in the
   refrigerator up to 24 hours.

KEY INGREDIENT: Wild Blueberries

Wild blueberries contain more of the powerful antioxidant anthocyanin than cultivated blueberries do, so it's worth seeking them out and adding them to your rotation. Most well-stocked supermarkets will have wild blueberries in their frozen fruit section. In addition to the anti-inflammatory properties wild blueberries possess, anthocyanin is thought to play a role in brain and eye health. Wild blueberries also have 30 percent less (natural) sugar than cultivated blueberries have.

Although the starring role in this smoothie goes to the wild blueberries, that isn't the only ingredient working to reduce inflammation for you. This smoothie brings additional anti-inflammatory goodness through flaxseeds, parsley, ginger, and almonds. It's aptly named a *power smoothie*!

Per Serving
Calories: 216 | Fat: 9.7 g | Protein: 5.6 g | Sodium: 10 mg
Fiber: 6.6 g | Carbohydrates: 28.7 g | Sugar: 14.7 g

CHOCOLATE CHERRY SMOOTHIE

Serves 1

INGREDIENTS

¾ cup unsweetened almond milk, frozen

¾ cup unsweetened almond milk

1 cup cherries, pitted and frozen

1 tablespoon raw cacao powder

¼ teaspoon pure stevia powder

1 Place all ingredients in a large blender.

2 Blend the ingredients on high until thoroughly combined and smooth.

3 For ultimate thickness, consume immediately. Smoothie may also be stored in an airtight container in the refrigerator up to 24 hours.

KEY INGREDIENT: Cherries

Frozen pitted cherries are readily available in many supermarkets year-round. Cherries contain the antioxidants anthocyanin and cyanidin, which have anti-inflammatory effects. Cyanidin is regarded as one of the strongest antioxidants, and it quickly neutralizes reactive oxygen species. Thus, it has a powerful anti-inflammatory effect. It has been found to be especially helpful in dealing with inflammation associated with arthritis. In addition, cherries are a good source of fiber, potassium, calcium, vitamin A, and folic acid.

This is a thick and creamy smoothie that tastes more indulgent than it actually is. Freezing half of the almond milk helps create a thicker, more shake-like smoothie. You can do this easily in ice cube trays.

If you have trouble finding raw cacao powder, unsweetened cocoa powder is a good substitute. Although the antioxidants are diminished, it still has some anti-inflammatory properties.

Per Serving
Calories: 136 | Fat: 5.1 g | Protein: 3.7 g | Sodium: 270 mg
Fiber: 4.9 g | Carbohydrates: 24.5 g | Sugar: 15.4 g

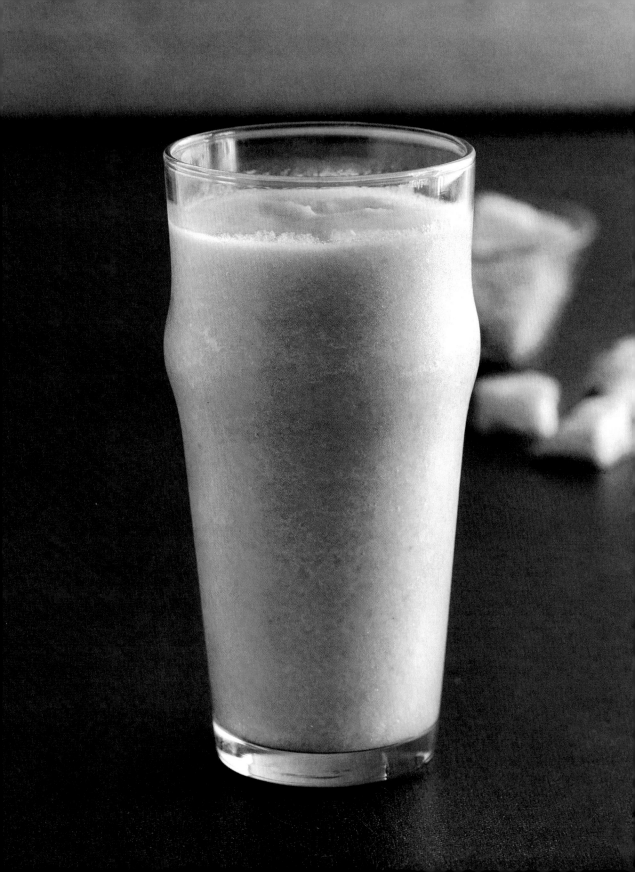

TURMERIC SMOOTHIE

Serves 1

INGREDIENTS

For the Turmeric Paste
¼ cup turmeric powder
½ cup water
¾ teaspoon black pepper

For the Smoothie
1 cup frozen pineapple chunks
1 cup frozen mango chunks
1–1½ cups cold water
1 teaspoon coconut oil
1 teaspoon peeled, chopped fresh ginger
1 teaspoon prepared turmeric paste

---

1 First, prepare the Turmeric Paste: Mix the turmeric powder and water in a small saucepan over low heat, stirring until a paste is formed.

2 Once you have a paste, stir in the black pepper. This recipe provides more than you'll need for this smoothie, so cool and store in a glass jar in the refrigerator up to 2 weeks.

3 Next, place all smoothie ingredients in a large blender.

4 Blend the ingredients on high until thoroughly combined and smooth.

5 Consume immediately or store in an airtight container in the refrigerator up to 24 hours.

KEY INGREDIENT: Turmeric

Turmeric is the all-star that gives this anti-inflammatory smoothie its gorgeous golden hue. Turmeric has over two dozen anti-inflammatory compounds, making it a very powerful ingredient to include in your diet. Turmeric has six different compounds that inhibit the COX-2 enzyme (a known promoter of inflammation). Curcumin is the most-noted compound in turmeric and is well known for its ability to ease arthritis pain. In fact, it has been shown to outperform many pharmaceuticals! In addition to the turmeric, you'll also get anti-inflammatory effects from the pineapple and fresh ginger in this smoothie. This is a sweet and spicy smoothie that is irresistible!

Turmeric is best absorbed when paired with black pepper, which is why pepper is included in the paste recipe. And you can use this turmeric paste in more than just this smoothie—try adding it to your scrambled eggs or favorite stir-fry as well!

Per Serving
Calories: 227 | Fat: 4.9 g | Protein: 2.6 g | Sodium: 2 mg
Fiber: 5.6 g | Carbohydrates: 48.5 g | Sugar: 38.8 g

AVOCADO-LADA SMOOTHIE

Serves 1

INGREDIENTS

1½ cups frozen pineapple chunks
½ medium avocado, peeled and pitted
2 cups baby spinach
3 tablespoons flaxseeds
1½ cups cold water

1   Place all ingredients in a large blender.

2   Blend the ingredients on high until thoroughly combined and smooth.

3   Consume immediately.

KEY INGREDIENT: Avocado

What could be better than enjoying the flavors of a piña colada in the health-promoting form of a smoothie? The avocado is one of the most nutrient-dense foods on the planet. Avocados have a very low glycemic index and are a great source of pantothenic acid; fiber; copper; folate; and vitamins K, B_6, E, and C. Their anti-inflammatory benefit comes from their fat content. They are a great source of omega-9 fatty acids (heart-healthy monounsaturated fats), which have been shown to improve insulin sensitivity and decrease inflammation.

Spinach, pineapple, and flaxseeds are also working in your favor with their anti-inflammatory compounds. This smoothie is excellent with plain water, or you could add a little extra natural sweetness with hydrating coconut water.

Per Serving
Calories: 414 | Fat: 22.0 g | Protein: 10.0 g | Sodium: 63 mg
Fiber: 17.8 g | Carbohydrates: 49.5 g | Sugar: 25.3 g

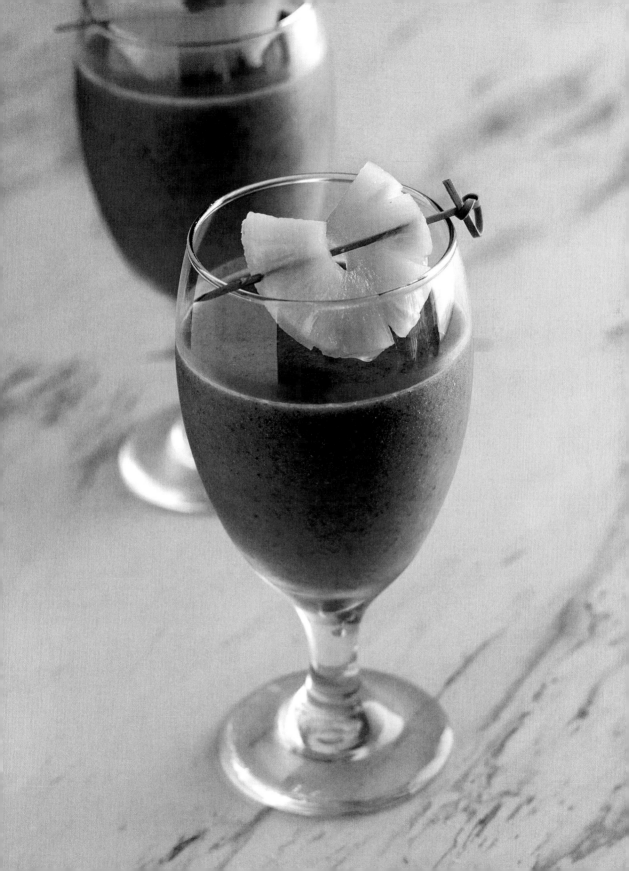

ALMOND FLAX SMOOTHIE

Serves 1

INGREDIENTS

1 large banana
⅓ cup ground flaxseed meal
1 cup unsweetened vanilla almond milk
1 tablespoon unsalted almond butter
¼ teaspoon ground cinnamon
1 cup ice

1 Place all ingredients in a large blender.
2 Blend the ingredients on high until thoroughly combined and smooth.
3 Consume immediately or store in an airtight container in the refrigerator up to 24 hours.

KEY INGREDIENT: Flaxseeds

Flaxseeds are an excellent source of the omega-3 fatty acid alpha-linolenic acid (ALA). ALA helps fight the damage in your body from free radicals and is also thought to improve insulin sensitivity. Studies have shown that people with chronic inflammation, especially those who are overweight, who supplement their diet with flaxseeds significantly lower the inflammation marker C-reactive protein.

Almonds, flaxseeds, and cinnamon all have anti-inflammatory properties. These ingredients just so happen to taste fantastic together as well! If you don't have almond butter on hand, you can easily make your own by blending whole almonds in a powerful blender or food processor. You may need to add a little oil to create a smooth butter.

Per Serving
Calories: 419 | Fat: 23.3 g | Protein: 13.6 g | Sodium: 182 mg
Fiber: 13.7 g | Carbohydrates: 42.6 g | Sugar: 15.5 g

VITAMIN C POWER SMOOTHIE

Serves 1

INGREDIENTS

½ medium banana, peeled and frozen
1 medium orange, peeled and cut into segments
1 medium kiwifruit, peeled and cut into quarters
2 cups baby spinach
¾ cup lite canned coconut milk
1 cup ice

1 Place all ingredients in a large blender.
2 Blend the ingredients on high until thoroughly combined and smooth.
3 Consume immediately.

KEY INGREDIENT: Kiwifruit

Kiwifruit contains enzymes that help break down inflammatory complexes in the body. In addition, kiwifruit has an antioxidant peptide, kissper, which is shown to effectively counteract oxidative stress and inflammatory responses in the body. Kiwifruit is also high in vitamin C, an immune boosting vitamin. In fact, you are getting a triple dose of vitamin C from the orange, kiwifruit, and spinach, making this a great smoothie to consume during the cold and flu season! The coconut milk gives this smoothie a creamy, tropical feel. Canned coconut milk is used here, and the lite variety helps keep calories in check.

Per Serving
Calories: 288 | Fat: 10.8 g | Protein: 4.2 g | Sodium: 60 mg
Fiber: 8.6 g | Carbohydrates: 45.4 g | Sugar: 27.5 g

AVOCADO CHOCOLATE SMOOTHIE

Serves 1

INGREDIENTS

½ medium banana

¼ medium avocado, peeled and pitted

1 cup vanilla almond milk

1 tablespoon unsalted almond butter

1 tablespoon raw cacao powder

¼ teaspoon pure stevia powder

½ cup ice

1 Place all ingredients in a large blender.

2 Blend the ingredients on high until thoroughly combined and smooth.

3 Consume immediately.

KEY INGREDIENT: Raw Cacao Powder

Cacao powder is made from unroasted cacao beans. It's easy to get cacao powder confused with cocoa powder, often used in baking, but they are different. While cocoa powder and cacao powder both start from the cacao bean, the difference is in the processing. The sharpest contrast is that cocoa powder is heated to very high temperatures. While this gives cocoa powder a less bitter taste, it also degrades its nutritional value. Cacao powder is processed at a very low heat, which helps it retain its enzymes, vitamins, and nutrients.

Cacao is rich in antioxidants. In fact, it ranks in the top twenty of all antioxidant foods, based on its Oxygen Radical Absorbance Capacity (ORAC) Scale—a test developed to measure the antioxidant capacity of foods. The powerful antioxidants in cacao, known as *flavonols*, are responsible for the anti-inflammatory effects it possesses. Flavonols can increase nitric oxide bioavailability and also activate nitric oxide synthase, an enzyme that helps the body produce nitric oxide. Nitric oxide is a signaling molecule that provides an anti-inflammatory effect in our bodies. This is why dark chocolate is known to be so healthful!

The banana, avocado, and almond butter also contribute to the nutrition of this smoothie. The best part, though, is that this smoothie gets the most amazing creamy texture from the avocado, and it tastes like a dreamy dessert!

Per Serving

Calories: 317 | Fat: 15.3 g | Protein: 6.7 g | Sodium: 154 mg
Fiber: 7.5 g | Carbohydrates: 38.2 g | Sugar: 23.0 g

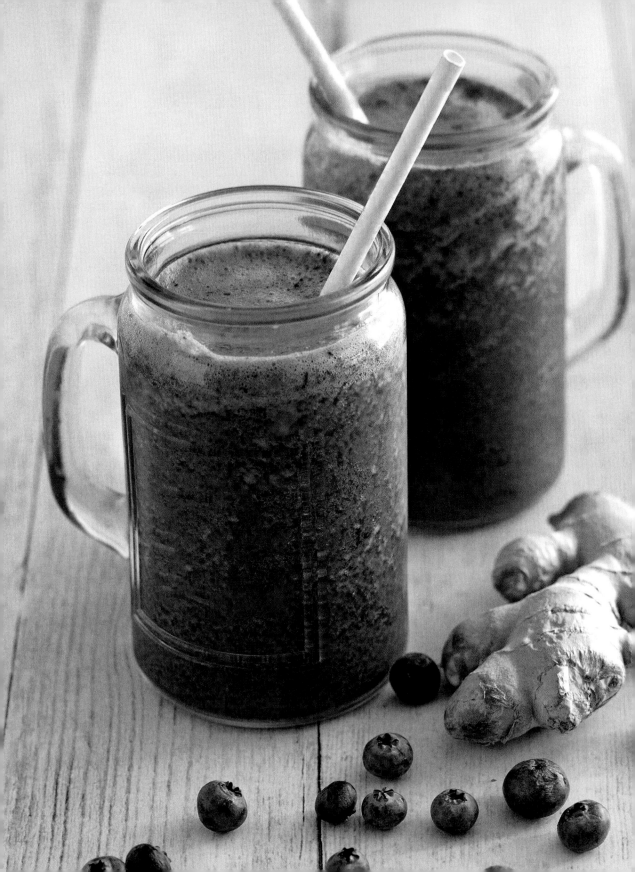

BLUEBERRY GINGER SMOOTHIE

Serves 2

INGREDIENTS

1 cup fresh blueberries

1 teaspoon peeled, chopped fresh ginger

1 cup unsweetened vanilla almond milk

1 cup sliced frozen banana

1 cup ice

---

1 Place all ingredients in a large blender.

2 Blend the ingredients on high until thoroughly combined and smooth.

3 Consume immediately or store in an airtight container in the refrigerator up to 24 hours.

KEY INGREDIENT: Blueberries

Blueberries are low in calories and high in antioxidants, and they give this smoothie a vibrant indigo color! Blueberries get their bright blue pigment from a class of antioxidants called *anthocyanins*, which fight inflammation. Anthocyanins have a positive effect on inflammation by inhibiting the expression and biological activity of some pro-inflammatory cytokines. Not only are blueberries going to help you fight inflammation, but they also have been linked to brain and heart health. They are powerful little berries!

The banana in this smoothie lends its natural sweetness. Frozen bananas give this smoothie extra creaminess, so make an effort to freeze the banana ahead of time. Simply slice your banana and freeze it in a freezer-safe container overnight. The fresh ginger adds zing, and ginger is another potent inflammation fighter!

Per Serving

Calories: 124 | Fat: 1.8 g | Protein: 1.9 g | Sodium: 91 mg
Fiber: 4.3 g | Carbohydrates: 29.0 g | Sugar: 16.8 g

CHOCOLATE ALMOND BUTTER SMOOTHIE

Serves 1

INGREDIENTS

1½ medium bananas, peeled and frozen

3 tablespoons unsweetened raw cacao powder

1 tablespoon unsalted almond butter

2 cups baby spinach

2 tablespoons ground flaxseed meal

1 cup unsweetened vanilla almond milk

1 cup ice

---

1 Place all ingredients in a large blender.

2 Blend the ingredients on high until thoroughly combined and smooth.

3 Consume immediately.

KEY INGREDIENT: Banana

Bananas are one of the most popular fruits, but they aren't often noted for their health benefits. Even so, they are a nutrient-dense food that has anti-inflammatory properties. Bananas have the anti-inflammatory antioxidant quercetin. In addition, bananas also contain the powerful flavonoid kaempferol. A diet high in kaempferol is correlated with reduced serum interleukin-6 levels, an inflammatory cytokine.

Almonds, spinach, cacao powder, and flaxseeds all bring anti-inflammatory properties to this smoothie. You're also getting a good amount of vitamin E, omega-3 fatty acids, and antioxidants in this drink.

Even though there's spinach in this smoothie, you'll only be able to focus on the lovely combination of chocolate and almond butter. The frozen bananas bring a creaminess and naturally sweeten the smoothie. If you like chocolate and peanut butter together, you'll love chocolate and almond butter! This is an anti-inflammatory smoothie that tastes like a treat.

Per Serving
Calories: 323 | Fat: 17.3 g | Protein: 12.7 g | Sodium: 228 mg
Fiber: 11.5 g | Carbohydrates: 33.7 g | Sugar: 8.6 g

PEACHY STRAWBERRY DESIRE SMOOTHIE

Serves 1

INGREDIENTS

1 cup frozen peaches
1 cup frozen strawberries
1 cup roughly chopped bok choy
1 cup unsweetened vanilla almond
  milk
¼ teaspoon pure vanilla extract
3 tablespoons hulled hemp seeds
¼ cup whole almonds
Handful of ice (optional)

1   Place all ingredients in a large
    blender.
2   Blend the ingredients on high
    until thoroughly combined and
    smooth.
3   Consume immediately.

KEY INGREDIENT: Bok Choy

Bok choy is one of those powerhouse vegetables that provides excellent anti-inflammatory benefits, but it isn't an ingredient you'd normally find in a smoothie. There's no reason why you shouldn't rotate the greens you use in smoothies, and bok choy is a particularly nutritious choice. Bok choy is loaded with vitamin A, vitamin C, manganese, and zinc. It also contains omega-3 fatty acids and alpha-linolenic acid (ALA), which works to keep chronic inflammation at bay. Bok choy also has a higher concentration of beta carotene and vitamin A than any other variety of cabbage.

Pair bok choy with frozen peaches and strawberries with vanilla extract, and you'll forget you're drinking such a healthy smoothie! Hemp seeds add some protein to this smoothie, and the whole almonds add to the anti-inflammatory power.

Per Serving
Calories: 530 | Fat: 34.5 g | Protein: 22.7 g | Sodium: 227 mg
Fiber: 12.6 g | Carbohydrates: 41.7 g | Sugar: 22.6 g

STRAWBERRY BANANA OATMEAL SMOOTHIE

Serves 1

INGREDIENTS

1 medium banana, peeled and frozen
1½ cups frozen strawberries
2 cups chopped romaine lettuce
¾ cup rolled oats
1 cup unsweetened vanilla almond
  milk

1   Place all ingredients in a large
    blender.
2   Blend the ingredients on high
    until thoroughly combined and
    smooth.
3   Consume immediately.

KEY INGREDIENT: Rolled Oats

Many people have heard that oats can help lower cholesterol numbers, but did you also know that oats can help reduce inflammation? It's true! Oats have special compounds called *avenanthramides*, which researchers believe play the biggest role in reducing inflammation. Avenanthramides are unique to oats and have been shown to reduce the inflammatory signals put out by the cells that line the blood vessels.

Even more, oats also have saponins, special phytochemicals that promote an anti-inflammatory environment systematically. This tasty smoothie also gets extra anti-inflammatory properties from the strawberries and romaine lettuce. Freeze your banana ahead of time for an extra-creamy smoothie. And using vanilla almond milk adds great flavor.

Per Serving
Calories: 513 | Fat: 8.8 g | Protein: 14.9 g | Sodium: 192 mg
Fiber: 18.2 g | Carbohydrates: 100.5 g | Sugar: 27.6 g

RASPBERRY LEMON TART SMOOTHIE

Serves 1

INGREDIENTS

1½ cups frozen raspberries
2 tablespoons fresh lemon juice
¾ cup water
½ teaspoon pure stevia powder

1 Place all ingredients in a large blender.

2 Blend the ingredients on high until thoroughly combined and smooth.

3 Consume immediately or store in an airtight container in the refrigerator up to 24 hours.

KEY INGREDIENT: Raspberries

The raspberry is truly a powerful berry. Raspberries have been shown to inhibit the production of the same enzymes that anti-inflammatory products like ibuprofen and aspirin do! Like blueberries, raspberries are also high in anthocyanins, which are shown to reduce chronic inflammation in the body. Raspberries have one of the highest antioxidant levels of any fruit, so they are one of the healthiest fruits you can consume. Oxidative stress in your body can lead to health problems like heart disease and diabetes, and the antioxidants in raspberries fight that cellular damage from free radicals.

This smoothie is reminiscent of sweet-tart candies, but in healthy smoothie form! If you like tart raspberry lemonade, you'll love this smoothie. The tart flavor is balanced by the natural sweetness of pure stevia powder.

Per Serving
Calories: 115 | Fat: 0.0 g | Protein: 2.6 g | Sodium: 2 mg
Fiber: 13.7 g | Carbohydrates: 27.2 g | Sugar: 10.1 g

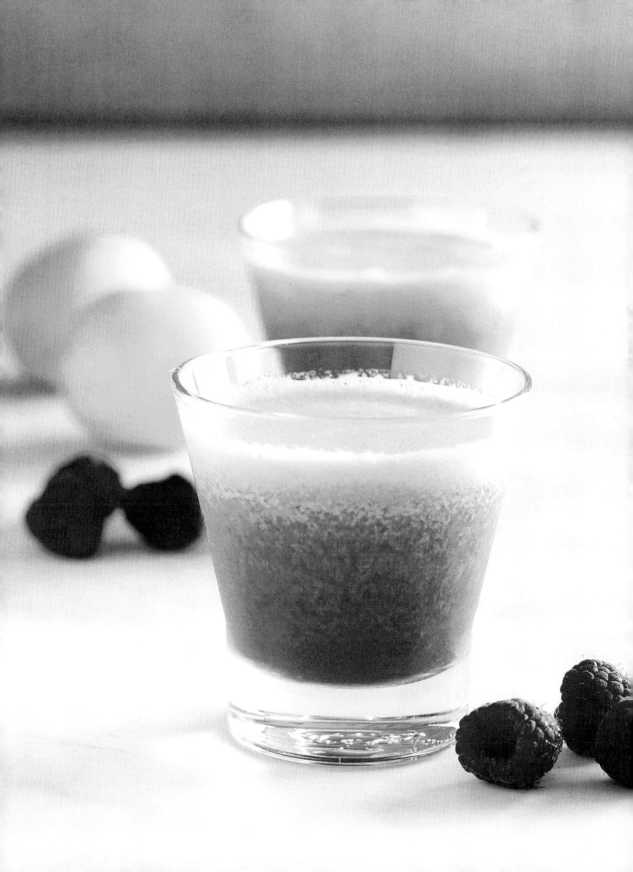

PEAR GINGER SMOOTHIE

Serves 1

INGREDIENTS

1 large ripe pear, cored and quartered

2 cups baby spinach

1 tablespoon peeled, chopped fresh ginger

1 tablespoon fresh lemon juice

¼ cup whole almonds

¾ cup cold water

1 cup ice

---

1 Place all ingredients in a large blender.

2 Blend the ingredients on high until thoroughly combined and smooth.

3 Consume immediately.

KEY INGREDIENT: Fresh Ginger

Pears and ginger go together naturally, and what a great way to incorporate the fantastic inflammation-fighting ginger into your smoothie. Ginger has a long history of medicinal use, dating back to ancient times, including use as a strong inflammation fighter. One group of compounds in ginger that are shown to have anti-inflammatory effects are gingerols. Gingerols inhibit the synthesis of pro-inflammatory cytokines.

Ginger also contains a protein-digesting enzyme called *zingibain*, which has also been shown to reduce inflammation in the body. This anti-inflammatory action makes ginger excellent for reducing pain after intense physical exercise. As a result, this juice, and all of the recipes with fresh ginger, are excellent as recovery drinks. Research has shown that the anti-inflammatory actions are equal to anti-inflammatory drugs, with patients reporting the same amount of pain relief when using ginger instead of over-the-counter drugs!

There are even more inflammation fighters in this smoothie, including the baby spinach and almonds. A pear has a lot of natural sugars, which gives this smoothie a subtle sweetness to offset the spicy ginger. Ginger brings a nice bite to smoothies. If you find it too strong, you can always use less and work your way up to the full recipe amount.

Per Serving

Calories: 334 | Fat: 17.2 g | Protein: 10.6 g | Sodium: 48 mg
Fiber: 11.4 g | Carbohydrates: 37.9 g | Sugar: 19.4 g

VA-VA-VA-VOOM ENERGY SMOOTHIE

Serves 1

INGREDIENTS

¼ medium avocado, peeled and pitted
1 medium Granny Smith apple, cored and quartered
½ medium cucumber
1 cup spinach
1 cup chopped romaine lettuce
1 cup chopped kale, veins removed
1 medium banana, peeled and frozen
2 tablespoons chia seeds
1 cup cold water
1 cup ice

1 Place all ingredients in a large blender.

2 Blend the ingredients on high until thoroughly combined and smooth.

3 Consume immediately.

KEY INGREDIENT: Spinach

Leafy green vegetables like spinach have potent antioxidants that have been shown to reduce inflammation. Spinach contains two carotenoids, lutein and zeaxanthin. Research has shown that the higher the levels of these two carotenoids are in the blood, the lower the inflammation markers will be. Spinach also contains flavonoids, powerful antioxidants that protect against free radical damage within your body. Spinach is also a good source of vitamins A and C, manganese, zinc, and selenium.

If you want your smoothie to fight inflammation *and* give you loads of energy, this is the smoothie for you. Packing three cups of greens into this smoothie will energize you and keep you going! It's a great idea to include a lot of greens in your diet every day, and smoothies like this make it an easy task.

Per Serving
Calories: 388 | Fat: 11.1 g | Protein: 8.8 g | Sodium: 41 mg
Fiber: 20.0 g | Carbohydrates: 67.4 g | Sugar: 33.0 g

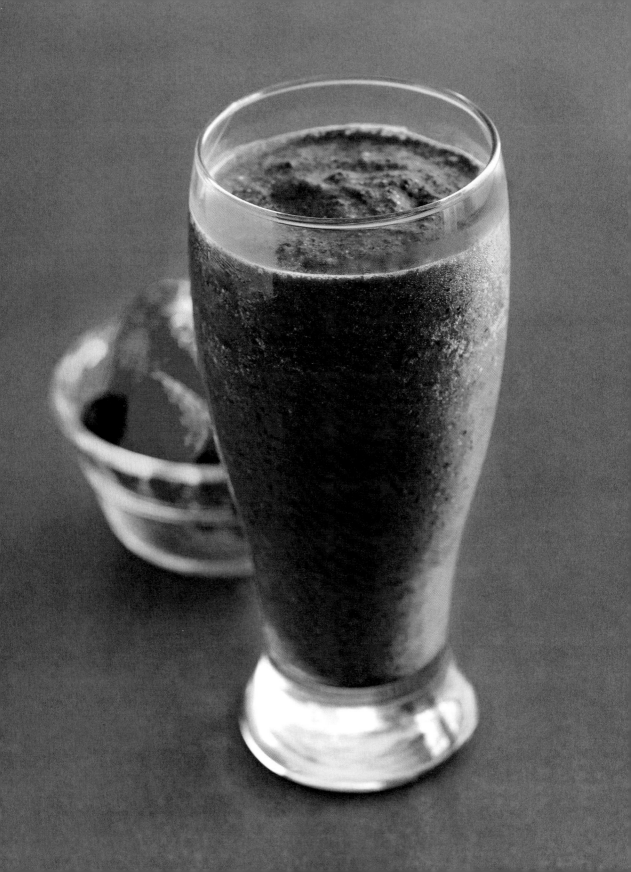

MIXED BERRY SMOOTHIE

Serves 2

INGREDIENTS

½ cup strawberry chunks
½ cup raspberries
½ cup blueberries
1 cup unsweetened vanilla almond
   milk
½ teaspoon pure vanilla extract

1 Place all ingredients in a large
   blender.

2 Blend the ingredients on high
   until thoroughly combined and
   smooth.

3 Consume immediately or store
   in an airtight container in the
   refrigerator up to 24 hours.

KEY INGREDIENT: Berries

Berries of all kinds have an anti-inflammatory effect, so why not triple up and put three of them in one powerful smoothie? Strawberries, raspberries, and blueberries, with their strong antioxidant profiles, bring their unique properties to this smoothie. All three berries are rich in flavonoids, which have been touted for their ability to block the production of molecules that promote inflammation, specifically the cyclooxygenase (COX) and lipoxygenase (LOX) enzymes.

Studies have shown that the plant compounds in berries can reduce the risk of serious diseases like cardiovascular disease and cancer. In addition to their anti-inflammatory properties, the three berries in this smoothie contain good amounts of vitamin C, vitamin K, manganese, folate, copper, and fiber!

Berries deliver great nutrition and taste delicious. This smoothie takes advantage of that flavor, which is complemented by a touch of vanilla.

Per Serving
Calories: 67 | Fat: 1.8 g | Protein: 1.4 g | Sodium: 90 mg
Fiber: 4.2 g | Carbohydrates: 13.4 g | Sugar: 7.4 g

TROPICAL GREEN SMOOTHIE

Serves 1

INGREDIENTS

1 cup frozen pineapple chunks
½ cup frozen mango chunks
1 medium ripe banana (frozen or not)
1 cup chopped kale, veins removed
3 tablespoons hemp seeds
1 cup cold unsweetened coconut
   water

1   Place all ingredients in a large
    blender.

2   Blend the ingredients on high
    until thoroughly combined and
    smooth.

3   Consume immediately.

KEY INGREDIENT: Pineapple

Pineapple is one of the sweetest fruits and therefore a great natural sweetener for both juices and smoothies. It can help offset the earthy or bitter flavor of many greens and make them more palatable. Pineapples are good for more than just their sweetening ability, though. They are also considered a powerful anti-inflammatory food because they contain bromelain. Bromelain is a protein-digesting enzyme that works similarly to anti-inflammatory drugs in the body. It is easily absorbed in the body without degrading or losing its biological activity. Research has shown that bromelain reduces pain and swelling, so it is especially helpful for athletic recovery, arthritis symptoms, or any type of physical trauma.

In addition to its anti-inflammatory action, bromelain has been shown to be helpful in a number of other conditions. Because it helps the body break down proteins, it's an excellent digestive aid. Research has shown that it even has a protective effect against cancer, cardiovascular disease, and diabetes. This powerful enzyme is what makes pineapple a smart dietary choice.

All of the sweet, tropical-tasting fruit in this smoothie totally masks the taste of the kale, so even the pickiest palates won't realize it's there. Hemp seeds add protein to this smoothie, which will help keep you full longer. Coconut water is hydrating and adds another tropical component. Plain water is a fine substitute if you don't have coconut water.

Per Serving
Calories: 458 | Fat: 15.2 g | Protein: 16.2 g | Sodium: 260 mg
Fiber: 10.9 g | Carbohydrates: 73.4 g | Sugar: 48.3 g

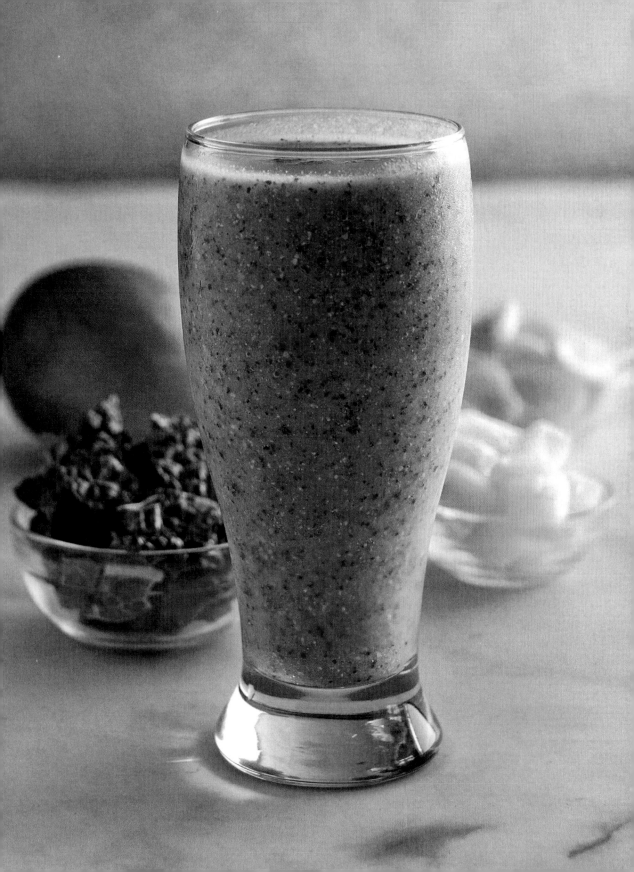

WAKE-ME-UP GREEN SMOOTHIE

Serves 1

INGREDIENTS

½ cup coconut water

Juice from 1 medium lime

1" piece fresh ginger, peeled and sliced

½ cup packed parsley

2 cups chopped kale, veins removed

1 medium Red Delicious apple, cut into chunks

½ medium banana

1 cup ice

1 Place all ingredients in a large blender.

2 Blend the ingredients on high until thoroughly combined and smooth.

3 Consume immediately.

KEY INGREDIENT: Lime

Citrus fruits such as lime are high in vitamin C, which provides protection against inflammation. Studies have found that moderate amounts of vitamin C can positively affect inflammation markers, reducing them significantly. Consuming lime juice is a great way to naturally increase your vitamin C intake.

This is the perfect smoothie to drink in the morning. Only lightly sweet, this is a smoothie that has a bite from the ginger, tartness from the lime, and a little bitterness from the greens. It tastes healthy and will make you feel healthy! It will quickly become one of your favorite ways to start the day.

Per Serving
Calories: 228 | Fat: 0.7 g | Protein: 4.4 g | Sodium: 156 mg
Fiber: 10.0 g | Carbohydrates: 54.2 g | Sugar: 33.7 g

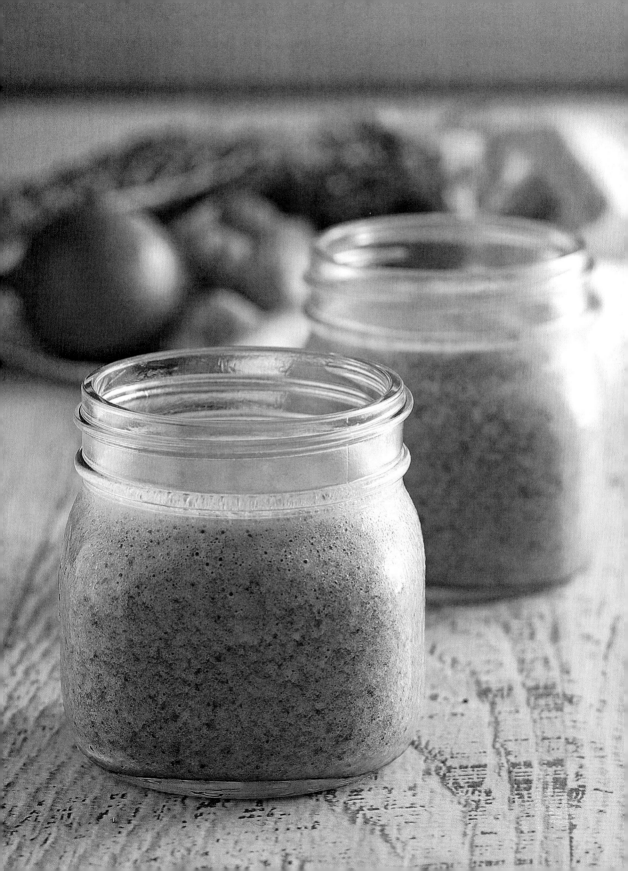

MANGO ZINGER SMOOTHIE

Serves 1

INGREDIENTS

1 cup frozen mango chunks

½" piece fresh ginger, peeled and cut
into chunks

1 medium banana, peeled and
frozen

2 cups spinach

1 cup unsweetened vanilla almond
milk

3 tablespoons chia seeds

1 tablespoon fresh lime juice

---

1   Place all ingredients in a large
    blender.

2   Blend the ingredients on high
    until thoroughly combined and
    smooth.

3   Consume immediately.

KEY INGREDIENT: Chia Seeds

Chia seeds are a good source of alpha-linolenic acid (ALA), an omega-3 fatty acid known for helping protect against inflammation. A number of studies have shown that increasing daily amounts of ALA helps reduce pain and joint pain in arthritis patients.

Chia seeds also contain quercetin, an anti-inflammatory antioxidant. Quercetin inhibits production of inflammation-producing enzymes in the body. In addition to being anti-inflammatory, quercetin has also been shown to have anticarcinogenic and antiviral properties.

Mangoes, spinach, ginger, limes, and almonds also have anti-inflammatory powers. Put all of these ingredients together, and you end up with a strong anti-inflammatory drink. You are going to love the texture frozen mango gives this smoothie.

Per Serving

Calories: 402 | Fat: 13.0 g | Protein: 10.6 g | Sodium: 233 mg
Fiber: 18.9 g | Carbohydrates: 70.6 g | Sugar: 37.9 g

Chapter 3

JUICES

Freshly juiced fruits and vegetables can add a tremendous amount of nutrients to your diet. While smoothies are made by blending the *whole* food, juices are made by extracting just the juice from the fruits and vegetables. Both are beneficial and have a place in a balanced, healthy diet.

You are able to consume more juice in one sitting than a smoothie because smoothies are more filling and caloric. Some people believe that juicing allows for quicker absorption of nutrients because the fiber is removed.

In order to make the juices in this chapter you'll need a juicer. Juicers are widely available in stores and online in every price range. The two types of juicers you'll find are centrifugal and masticating. The most economical of these two types are centrifugal juicers. Centrifugal juicers are higher-speed juicers, but they are not as efficient as the masticating style. A masticating juicer works at a slower speed and retains more of the vegetables' and fruits' nutrients. The juice from masticating juicers also lasts significantly longer than centrifugal juicers.

No matter which kind you choose, you'll find that making fresh juice at home is easy and delicious. Adding juicing to your daily routine is a surefire way to improve your health.

CARROT GINGER

Serves 1

INGREDIENTS

5 medium carrots
1 tablespoon peeled, coarsely
    chopped ginger

1 Prepare the carrots by chopping off the tops and tips and then cutting them into appropriate-sized pieces for your juicer.

2 Process the carrots and ginger through the juicer.

3 Strain through a fine-mesh sieve if desired.

4 Consume immediately over ice or allow to chill in the refrigerator before serving.

5 Can be stored in a glass airtight container in the refrigerator up to 12 hours if using a centrifugal juicer and up to 3 days if using a masticating juicer.

KEY INGREDIENT: Ginger

Ginger is so powerful because it contains a number of compounds that help fight inflammation. The gingerols in ginger have been shown to suppress the pro-inflammatory compounds cytokines and chemokines and fight off free radicals that can lead to inflammation. In addition to its anti-inflammatory benefits, ginger eases nausea, helps lower blood sugars, and protects against cardiovascular disease. The same compounds that fight inflammation have been shown to decrease glucose, total cholesterol, and triglycerides. Ginger also has antifungal properties, so it can help with related conditions, such as yeast infections and jock itch.

The sweet carrots in this juice recipe offset the spicy ginger. This is a great energizing juice that can help you get moving in the morning or get through an afternoon slump!

Per Serving
Calories: 109 | Fat: 0.5 g | Protein: 2.0 g | Sodium: 210 mg
Fiber: 0.0 g | Carbohydrates: 21.6 g | Sugar: 14.6 g

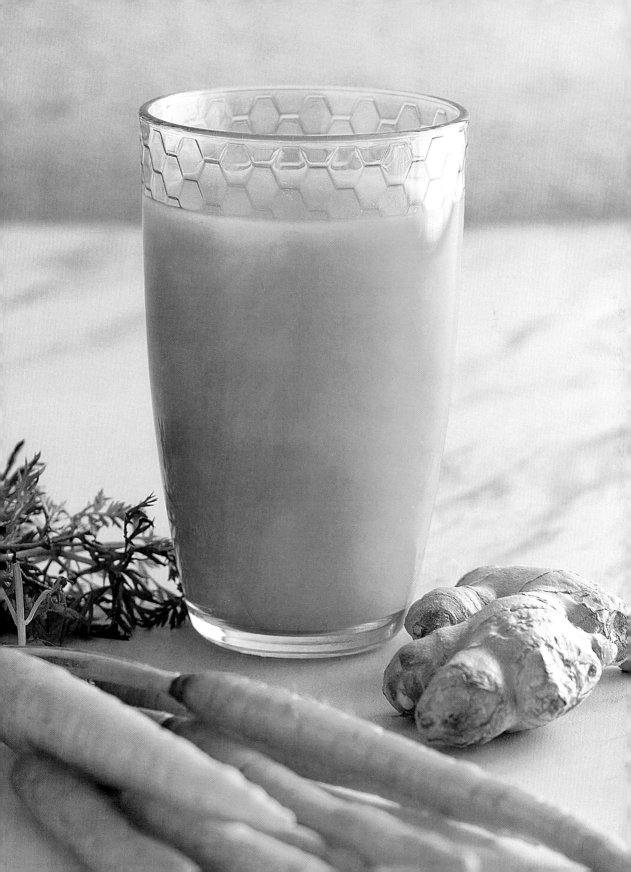

GREEN PINEAPPLE

Serves 2

INGREDIENTS

½ medium pineapple, peeled and cut into chunks
2 cups packed baby spinach

---

1 Process the pineapple and spinach through the juicer.

2 Strain through a fine-mesh sieve if desired.

3 Consume immediately over ice or allow to chill in the refrigerator before serving.

4 Can be stored in a glass airtight container in the refrigerator up to 12 hours if using a centrifugal juicer and up to 3 days if using a masticating juicer.

KEY INGREDIENT: Pineapple

In addition to containing the digestive enzyme bromelain, which has an anti-inflammatory effect, pineapples are packed with health-promoting nutrients. They are an excellent source of vitamin C and manganese and are also a great source of copper, vitamins B_6 and B_1, fiber, and folate. The vitamin C in pineapple helps your body fight free radical damage and helps keep inflammation at bay also.

Another bonus of consuming pineapple is that it may help your mental health. Pineapple is a good source of the amino acid tryptophan, which is used by the body to produce serotonin. Serotonin is the hormone associated with feelings of happiness and well-being. This green juice is sweet and loved by kids and adults alike.

Per Serving
Calories: 111 | Fat: 0.2 g | Protein: 2.1 g | Sodium: 25 mg
Fiber: 0.0 g | Carbohydrates: 26.9 g | Sugar: 22.4 g

POPEYE JUICE

Serves 2

INGREDIENTS

2 medium carrots
2 cups packed baby spinach
1 medium orange, peeled and
  segmented

1 Prepare the carrots by cutting off the tops and tips and cutting them into appropriate-sized pieces for your juicer.

2 Process the carrots, spinach, and orange through the juicer.

3 Strain through a fine-mesh sieve if desired.

4 Consume immediately over ice or allow to chill in the refrigerator before serving.

5 Can be stored in a glass airtight container in the refrigerator up to 12 hours if using a centrifugal juicer and up to 3 days if using a masticating juicer.

KEY INGREDIENT: Spinach

Spinach has a long list of health benefits; Popeye favored it for good reason! It's one of the most nutrient-dense foods you can consume. It packs in a wide range of vitamins and minerals, including vitamins A, C, K, E, B_2, and B_6; niacin; folate; calcium; copper; iron; and manganese. That's just a partial list of the important nutrients found in this leafy green vegetable!

All of those nutrients contribute to spinach having a host of health benefits. Spinach gets its anti-inflammatory powers, in part, thanks to its high vitamin K content, which has been shown to suppress the production of pro-inflammatory cytokines. High vitamin K intake is also associated with low concentrations of several pro-inflammatory biomarkers.

In addition to the vitamin K, spinach also contains two unique carotenoids, neoxanthin and violaxanthin, that help fight inflammation. These two carotenoids are thought to reduce inflammation in the digestive tract after the consumption of spinach.

Per Serving
Calories: 58 | Fat: 0.2 g | Protein: 2.0 g | Sodium: 65 mg
Fiber: 0.0 g | Carbohydrates: 11.5 g | Sugar: 9.9 g

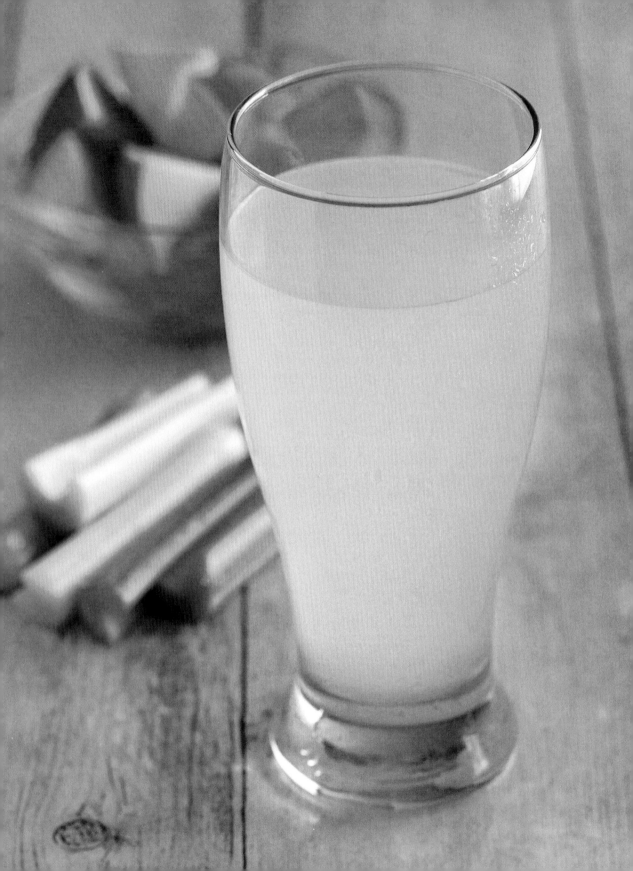

CELERY SUNSHINE

Serves 1

INGREDIENTS

2 medium stalks celery
3 medium apples
1 medium lemon, peeled and
    segmented

1   Prepare the celery stalks
    by cutting them into the
    appropriate-sized pieces for
    your juicer.

2   Prepare the apples by coring
    them and cutting them into
    appropriate-sized pieces for
    your juicer.

3   Process the celery, apples, and
    lemon through the juicer.

4   Consume immediately over ice
    or allow to chill in the refrigera-
    tor before serving.

5   Can be stored in a glass air-
    tight container in the refriger-
    ator up to 12 hours if using a
    centrifugal juicer and up to
    3 days if using a masticating
    juicer.

KEY INGREDIENT: Celery

Celery is well known as a low-calorie food with a high water content. Oh, but there's so much more to this crunchy vegetable. While it's a good source of vitamin C, more than a dozen other antioxidants have also been identified in celery.

Its wide range of protective antioxidants is what makes celery a standout nutritionally. Celery contains a class of antioxidants known as *phenolic acids*. Phenolic acids have protective qualities and fight inflammation. It's been found that these antioxidants inhibit protein denaturation, which is associated with increased inflammation. Consumption of celery juice has been studied and found to have an anti-inflammatory effect by decreasing levels of pro-inflammatory cytokines.

While celery juice alone isn't the most palatable juice, when combined with apples and lemon, it's quite refreshing. This juice is the color of sunshine and is sure to brighten any morning.

Per Serving
Calories: 275 | Fat: 0.6 g | Protein: 1.6 g | Sodium: 70 mg
Fiber: 0.0 g | Carbohydrates: 67.0 g | Sugar: 59.3 g

SWEET PARSLEY

Serves 2
INGREDIENTS

1 cup packed parsley leaves
3 cups seedless purple grapes

---

1 Process parsley and grapes through the juicer.

2 Strain through a fine-mesh sieve if desired.

3 Consume immediately over ice or allow to chill in the refrigerator before serving.

4 Can be stored in a glass airtight container in the refrigerator up to 12 hours if using a centrifugal juicer and up to 3 days if using a masticating juicer.

KEY INGREDIENT: Parsley

Parsley is a wholly underrated herb. It may be an afterthought in recipes or used only as garnish by some, but it deserves much more attention. Parsley comes with a whole range of health benefits that are not insignificant. Parsley contains myricetin, which is a potent anticancer compound and also fights diabetes. Parsley can also help you combat bad breath, which is important even if it's not as serious! It's also worth noting that parsley is high in vitamin C and vitamin A.

Parsley is also an outstanding herb for its anti-inflammatory properties. Parsley contains the flavonoid apigenin, which has been studied for its anti-inflammation effects. It was found that apigenin inhibited the collagenase activity present in rheumatoid arthritis. Like spinach, parsley is also high in vitamin K, which been shown to suppress the production of pro-inflammatory cytokines.

Take a second look at parsley; it's more than just a pretty garnish!

Per Serving
Calories: 156 | Fat: 0.4 g | Protein: 1.5 g | Sodium: 21 mg
Fiber: 0.0 g | Carbohydrates: 39.9 g | Sugar: 35.3 g

KALE-ING IT

Serves 2

INGREDIENTS

2 medium carrots
1 medium apple
3 large kale leaves, veins removed
½ medium pineapple, peeled and
  cut into chunks

1 Prepare the carrots by cutting off the tops and tips and cutting them into appropriate-sized pieces for your juicer.

2 Prepare the apple by coring and cutting into appropriate-sized pieces for your juicer.

3 Process the kale leaves, carrots, apple, and pineapple through the juicer.

4 Strain through a fine-mesh sieve if desired.

5 Consume immediately over ice or allow to chill in the refrigerator before serving.

6 Can be stored in a glass airtight container in the refrigerator up to 12 hours if using a centrifugal juicer and up to 3 days if using a masticating juicer.

KEY INGREDIENT: Kale

Kale has recently enjoyed a rise to popularity, and for good reason. This leafy green vegetable has a lot of goodness hiding in those leaves. Kale is high in vitamin K, vitamin A, vitamin C, vitamin B_6, manganese, copper, and iron. In fact, calorie for calorie, kale is higher in iron than beef is! Over forty-five different flavonoids have been discovered in kale, which help to make it a potent anticancer food.

Two nutrients in particular help kale with its inflammation-fighting power: vitamin K and the omega-3 fatty acid alpha-linolenic acid (ALA). Vitamin K can suppress the production of pro-inflammatory cytokines. ALA acts as an antioxidant and suppresses the production of inflammation-causing myeloperoxidase in the body.

While by itself kale may not be the best-tasting vegetable, in this juice it is amply sweetened by carrots, apple, and pineapple. This juice is an excellent way to enjoy the health benefits from kale.

Per Serving
Calories: 173 | Fat: 0.4 g | Protein: 1.7 g | Sodium: 50 mg
Fiber: 0.0 g | Carbohydrates: 41.9 g | Sugar: 35.0 g

BLACKBERRY SENSATION

Serves 1

INGREDIENTS

1 large apple
2 cups ripe blackberries

---

1 Prepare the apple by coring it and cutting it into appropriate-sized pieces for your juicer.

2 Process the apple and blackberries through juicer.

3 Strain with a fine-mesh sieve if desired.

4 Consume immediately over ice or allow to chill in the refrigerator before serving.

5 Can be stored in a glass airtight container in the refrigerator up to 12 hours if using a centrifugal juicer and up to 3 days if using a masticating juicer.

KEY INGREDIENT: Blackberry

It's a beautiful thing when delicious food also happens to have incredible nutritional qualities. That's the case with the splendid blackberry. Blackberries are a tasty fruit that rank highly on nutritional charts.

Like all berries, blackberries are blessed with an abundance of antioxidants. Blackberries contain high levels of anthocyanins and other phenolic compounds, mainly flavonols and ellagitannins. Ellagitannins have been established to have strong anti-inflammatory effects in the body, even though the mechanisms aren't totally clear. It is known that foods with high levels of antioxidants contribute to reduced oxidative stress from free radicals in the body, which can result in anti-inflammatory activity.

This juice is vibrantly hued, perfectly sweet, and pairs perfectly with your breakfast meal.

Per Serving
Calories: 166 | Fat: 1.1 g | Protein: 1.5 g | Sodium: 3 mg
Fiber: 0.0 g | Carbohydrates: 33.2 g | Sugar: 33.0 g

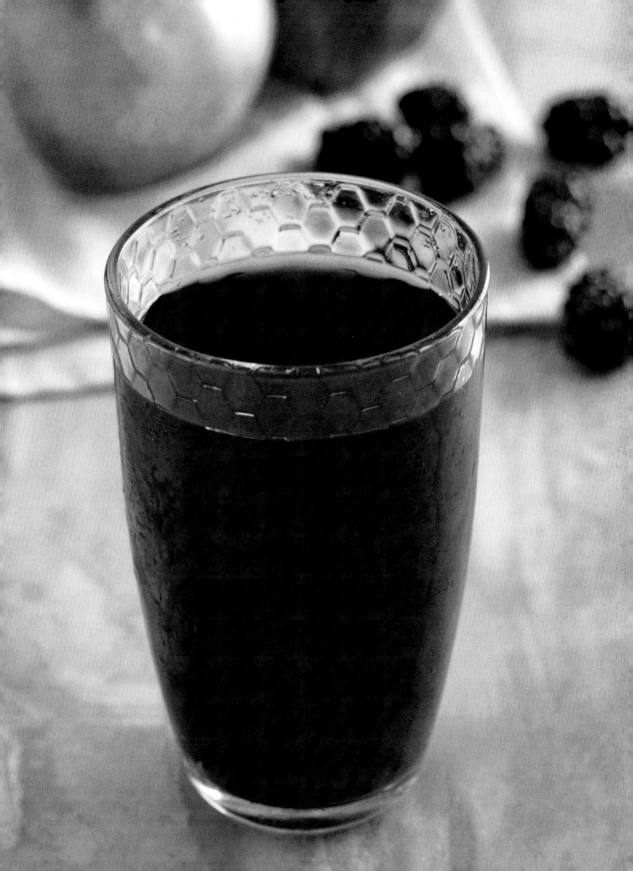

MINT REFRESHER

Serves 1

INGREDIENTS

1 large cucumber
¾ cup mint leaves

1 Prepare the cucumber by cutting off and discarding the ends and cutting the cucumber into appropriate-sized pieces for your juicer.

2 Process the cucumber and mint leaves through the juicer.

3 Strain with a fine-mesh sieve if desired.

4 Consume immediately over ice or allow to chill in the refrigerator before serving.

5 Can be stored in a glass airtight container in the refrigerator up to 12 hours if using a centrifugal juicer and up to 3 days if using a masticating juicer.

KEY INGREDIENT: Mint

Ah, mint. It's a refreshing herb that brings fresh flavor to any dish or drink. It's also loaded with health benefits. Mint is used to treat a variety of ailments, including digestive upset, headaches, dandruff, nausea, and skin conditions. It inhibits the growth of many different bacteria. Mint is also a stimulant, providing a natural energy boost.

Mint has traditionally been consumed as an anti-inflammatory for the lungs. Studies have been conducted that show promise that mint may be used to treat asthma in the future. One of mint's powerful nutrients, rosmarinic acid, was found to block inflammatory action in the body.

This juice is light and refreshing. For a stronger mint flavor, you can use a full cup of mint leaves. In addition to this refreshing juice, try adding mint leaves to your favorite salad or infuse your water with fresh mint leaves.

Per Serving
Calories: 48 | Fat: 0.3 g | Protein: 1.7 g | Sodium: 11 mg
Fiber: 0.0 g | Carbohydrates: 10.8 g | Sugar: 5.0 g

SWEET BROCCOLI

Serves 2

INGREDIENTS

2 cups pineapple chunks (about ½ medium pineapple)

1 large orange, peeled and segmented

1 cup broccoli florets

1   Process the pineapple, orange, and broccoli through juicer.

2   Strain through a fine-mesh sieve if desired.

3   Consume immediately over ice or allow to chill in the refrigerator before serving.

4   Can be stored in a glass airtight container in the refrigerator up to 12 hours if using a centrifugal juicer and up to 3 days if using a masticating juicer.

KEY INGREDIENT: Broccoli

Broccoli has a number of different anti-inflammatory compounds. The sulfur-containing substance in broccoli, glucosinolate, is shown to lower levels of C-reactive protein, which is a blood protein used to measure the level of inflammation in the body.

Broccoli has three different kinds of antioxidants, making it one of the top vegetables you can consume for its nutritional benefit. It fights inflammation, has anticancer properties, helps your body with natural detoxification, and has also been shown to help lower blood cholesterol levels.

Juicing broccoli is an excellent way to reap its nutritional benefits, and doing so with sweet fruits like pineapple and orange makes it taste great.

Per Serving
Calories: 117 | Fat: 0.2 g | Protein: 1.7 g | Sodium: 16 mg
Fiber: 0.0 g | Carbohydrates: 28.1 g | Sugar: 13.9 g

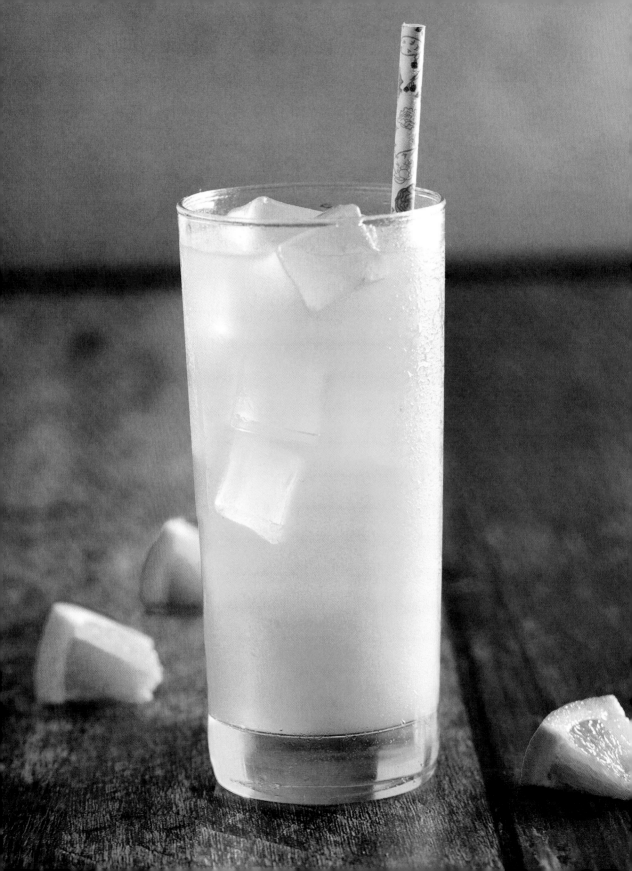

CITRUS CRUSH

Serves 1

INGREDIENTS

1 medium pink or red grapefruit, peeled and segmented

2 medium oranges, peeled and segmented

---

1 Process the grapefruit and oranges through the juicer.

2 Strain through a fine-mesh sieve if desired.

3 Consume immediately over ice or allow to chill in the refrigerator before serving.

4 Can be stored in a glass airtight container in the refrigerator up to 12 hours if using a centrifugal juicer and up to 3 days if using a masticating juicer.

KEY INGREDIENT: Grapefruit

Grapefruit is low in calories yet has impressive nutritional stats. It's an especially good source of vitamin C, which plays an important role in fighting inflammation. It's also a strong antioxidant that protects the body from free radicals, which have a pro-inflammatory effect. Vitamin C supplementation has been found to protect against certain diseases like coronary heart disease and gout, both of which have inflammatory components. The orange in this juice recipe adds even more vitamin C. This grapefruit and orange combo is also a great immune-system booster.

Grapefruit has a number of other health benefits as well. It's been shown to be great for your skin, help reduce your risk of developing kidney stones, and boost your metabolism.

This is an eye-opening juice recipe that's terrific in the morning.

Per Serving

Calories: 298 | Fat: 0.6 g | Protein: 1.9 g | Sodium: 1 mg
Fiber: 0.0 g | Carbohydrates: 72.2 g | Sugar: 61.5 g

DRINK YOUR SALAD

Serves 2

INGREDIENTS

1 medium head romaine lettuce
2 large carrots
1 medium cucumber
2 large lemons, peeled and
  segmented

---

1   Prepare the romaine by
    removing the core and chop-
    ping it roughly.

2   Prepare the carrots by remov-
    ing the tops and tips and
    cutting them into appropriate-
    sized pieces for your juicer.

3   Prepare the cucumber by
    cutting off and discarding the
    ends and cutting the cucum-
    ber into appropriate-sized
    pieces for your juicer.

4   Process the romaine, car-
    rots, cucumber, and lemons
    through the juicer.

5   Strain through a fine-mesh
    sieve if desired.

6   Consume immediately over ice
    or allow to chill in the refrigera-
    tor before serving.

7   Can be stored in a glass air-
    tight container in the refriger-
    ator up to 12 hours if using a
    centrifugal juicer and up to
    3 days if using a masticating
    juicer.

KEY INGREDIENT: Romaine Lettuce

Romaine is a nutrient-dense leafy green vegetable. It's an excellent source of vitamins K and A and folate. Vitamin A has been shown to reduce inflammation and oxidative stress, and 2 cups of romaine lettuce, at just 16 calories, provides almost half of your daily requirement.

You'll also find a good amount of fiber, manganese, copper, vitamin B_1, vitamin B_2, iron, potassium, and vitamin C in romaine leaves. All of the vitamins and antioxidants in romaine lettuce can help boost your immune system, prevent signs of aging, promote healthy eyesight, and prevent cancer.

This juice is like eating a big salad, but in this juice version, nutrients are more quickly absorbed.

Per Serving
Calories: 80 | Fat: 0.9 g | Protein: 2.0 g | Sodium: 71 mg
Fiber: 0.0 g | Carbohydrates: 16.3 g | Sugar: 10.6 g

DEEP ORANGE

Serves 2

INGREDIENTS

2 large carrots
2 medium oranges, peeled and
    segmented

1   Prepare the carrots by removing the tops and tips. Cut into appropriate-sized pieces for your juicer.

2   Process the carrots and oranges through the juicer.

3   Strain through a fine-mesh sieve if desired.

4   Consume immediately over ice or allow to chill in the refrigerator before serving.

5   Can be stored in a glass airtight container in the refrigerator up to 12 hours if using a centrifugal juicer and up to 3 days if using a masticating juicer.

KEY INGREDIENT: Orange

Orange juice is one of the most popular juices on the planet. It turns out, if you love orange juice, that's a good thing, as it's helping you fight inflammation. Research suggests that some flavonoids found in oranges, such as hesperidin and naringenin, help suppress inflammatory responses in the body. Oranges also contain carotenoids, which have been shown to inhibit certain inflammatory responses. Furthering their inflammation-fighting powers even more, oranges also contain beta-cryptoxanthin, a phytochemical that has been shown to decrease the development of inflammatory joint conditions.

You can always juice plain oranges, but why not add carrots to the mix and increase the nutritional value? Carrots add even more vitamins and antioxidants to your glass of juice, and they are a naturally sweet vegetable!

Per Serving
Calories: 87 | Fat: 0.2 g | Protein: 1.7 g | Sodium: 49 mg
Fiber: 0.0 g | Carbohydrates: 18.7 g | Sugar: 17.2 g

OVER THE RAINBOW

Serves 3

INGREDIENTS

7 large rainbow chard leaves
2 medium apples
2 cups seedless purple grapes
1 cup pineapple chunks (about ¼
   medium pineapple)

1   Prepare rainbow chard by
    chopping the leaves and stem
    to appropriate-sized pieces for
    your juicer.

2   Prepare apples by coring and
    cutting them into appropriate-
    sized pieces for your juicer.

3   Process the rainbow chard,
    apples, grapes, and pineapple
    through the juicer.

4   Strain through a fine-mesh
    sieve if desired.

5   Consume immediately over ice
    or allow to chill in the refrigera-
    tor before serving.

6   Can be stored in a glass air-
    tight container in the refriger-
    ator up to 12 hours if using a
    centrifugal juicer and up to
    3 days if using a masticating
    juicer.

KEY INGREDIENT: Rainbow Chard

Rainbow chard is a variety of Swiss chard with vibrantly colored stalks. That color is thanks, in part, to the concentration of betalains present. These phytonutrients have been shown to suppress pro-inflammatory enzymes cyclooxygenase (COX) and lipoxygenase (LOX). Swiss chard also contains flavonoids like quercetin and kaempferol, which act as antihistamines and reduce allergic reactions and inflammatory responses in the body. All of these compounds acting together make rainbow chard an excellent anti-inflammatory food to include in your diet.

In addition, Swiss chard is one of the most vitamin- and mineral-rich green vegetables. It has been shown to be an excellent food for blood sugar regulation and cardiovascular health.

The apples, grapes, and pineapple work together to mellow out the stronger flavor associated with the rainbow chard, making this a tasty and nutritious juice recipe.

Per Serving
Calories: 159 | Fat: 0.4 g | Protein: 1.4 g | Sodium: 241 mg
Fiber: 0.0 g | Carbohydrates: 40.0 g | Sugar: 34.8 g

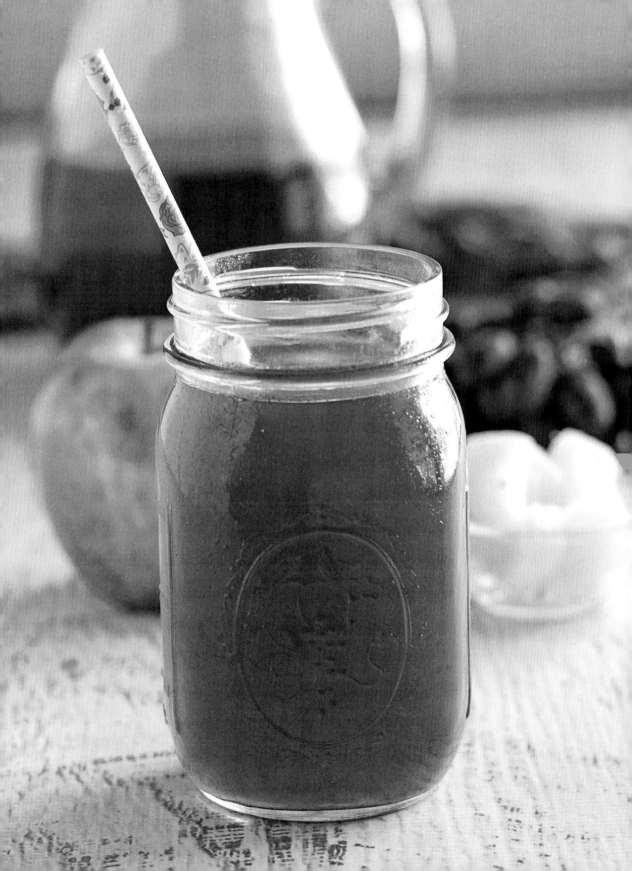

QUADRUPLE THREAT

Serves 1

INGREDIENTS

3 large collard greens leaves
1 cup seedless purple grapes
1 cup pineapple chunks (about ¼
  medium pineapple)
1 tablespoon peeled, chopped fresh
  ginger

---

1 Prepare the collard greens by removing and discarding the tough stem and roughly chopping the leaves.

2 Process all ingredients through the juicer.

3 Strain with a fine-mesh sieve if desired.

4 Consume immediately over ice or allow to chill in the refrigerator before serving.

5 Can be stored in a glass airtight container in the refrigerator up to 12 hours if using a centrifugal juicer and up to 3 days if using a masticating juicer.

KEY INGREDIENT: Collard Greens

Collard greens are an excellent source of two key nutrients that are known to fight inflammation: vitamin K and alpha-linolenic acid (ALA). In addition to these two key components, collard greens also contain glucobrassicin. Glucobrassicin can be easily converted into indole-3-carbinol. This is significant because indole-3-carbinol can prevent inflammatory responses at a very early stage.

Another important thing to know about collard greens is that they contain a peptide called glutathione. This helps the liver cleanse, protects against cancer, and boosts immune function. In fact, it is believed that the levels of glutathione in our blood can be a predictor of how long a person will live!

This juice recipe is called Quadruple Threat because four potent foods are working together to fight inflammation. Collard greens get help from the grapes, pineapple, and ginger here.

Per Serving
Calories: 176 | Fat: 0.6 g | Protein: 1.4 g | Sodium: 22 mg
Fiber: 0.0 g | Carbohydrates: 47.8 g | Sugar: 40.2 g

PURPLE POWER

Serves 2

INGREDIENTS

¼ small head purple cabbage
3 cups seedless purple grapes

1 Prepare the cabbage by removing the core and cutting the ¼ of the head into appropriate-sized pieces for your juicer.

2 Process the cabbage and grapes through the juicer.

3 Strain with a fine-mesh sieve if desired.

4 Consume immediately over ice or allow to chill in the refrigerator before serving.

5 Can be stored in a glass airtight container in the refrigerator up to 12 hours if using a centrifugal juicer and up to 3 days if using a masticating juicer.

KEY INGREDIENT: Purple Cabbage

Cabbage is a cruciferous vegetable that contains sulforaphane. This compound makes red cabbage a potent inflammation killer. Sulforaphane regulates inflammation by altering the messaging molecules within the inflammatory system in the body. This also has a potent anticancer effect.

There are other nutrients in red cabbage that help control inflammation. Red cabbage contains thirty-six of the flavonoids known as anthocyanins, well-documented inflammation fighters known to reduce inflammation markers in the bloodstream. Cabbage is also an excellent source of vitamin K, which suppresses production of pro-inflammatory cytokines.

Cabbage has a mild bitter flavor, but when paired with sweet purple grapes, it is milder and easier to drink. The purple color of both these deeply hued ingredients makes a vibrant juice.

Per Serving
Calories: 166 | Fat: 0.3 g | Protein: 1.6 g | Sodium: 23 mg
Fiber: 0.0 g | Carbohydrates: 42.7 g | Sugar: 37.8 g

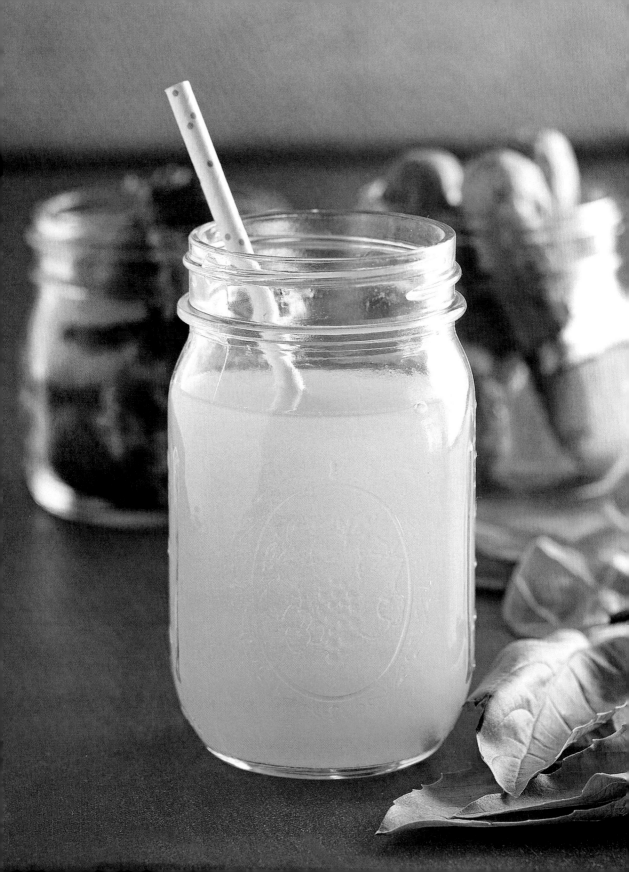

BASIL SMASH

Serves 1

INGREDIENTS

1 large cucumber
7 large strawberries, hulled
1 cup loosely packed basil leaves

---

1   Prepare the cucumber by cutting off and discarding the ends and cutting the cucumber into appropriate-sized pieces for your juicer.

2   Process all ingredients through the juicer.

3   Strain with a fine-mesh sieve if desired.

4   Consume immediately over ice or allow to chill in the refrigerator before serving.

5   Can be stored in a glass airtight container in the refrigerator up to 12 hours if using a centrifugal juicer and up to 3 days if using a masticating juicer.

KEY INGREDIENT: Basil

Basil is a beloved herb that provides lovely flavor in a variety of cooking applications. It just so happens to have anti-inflammatory properties, making it a wise choice to add to your anti-inflammatory drinks! Basil contains essential oils, such as eugenol, citronellol, and linalool. These essential oils are known to be enzyme-inhibiting oils, which help keep inflammation under control. Eugenol actually mimics the action of over-the-counter anti-inflammatory medications!

Studies have also shown that basil may have the ability to act as an adaptogen, helping your body react to stress and protect against the body's response to stressful environments.

The basil in this juice recipe pairs nicely with strawberry and cucumber, making this a lovely, refreshing spring or summer beverage.

Per Serving
Calories: 73 | Fat: 0.6 g | Protein: 1.6 g | Sodium: 7 mg
Fiber: 0.0 g | Carbohydrates: 16.8 g | Sugar: 11.3 g

GREEN MONSTER

Serves 2

INGREDIENTS

1 medium cucumber
2 stalks celery
1 bunch parsley, chopped roughly
2 medium limes, peeled and
  segmented
2 medium kiwifruits, peeled and
  chopped

---

1 Prepare the cucumber and celery stalks by cutting off and discarding the ends and then cutting the remaining portions into appropriate-sized pieces for your juicer.

2 Process the cucumber, celery, parsley, limes, and kiwifruits through the juicer.

3 Strain through a fine-mesh sieve if desired.

4 Consume immediately over ice or allow to chill in the refrigerator before serving.

5 Can be stored in a glass airtight container in the refrigerator up to 12 hours if using a centrifugal juicer and up to 3 days if using a masticating juicer.

KEY INGREDIENT: Parsley

Parsley is a rich source of flavonoids; folic acid; and vitamins A, C, and K. Looking closely at its anti-inflammatory properties, you can see it has more than one of its components at work. Parsley contains volatile oils, including myristicin, eugenol, limonene, and alpha-thujene. All of these oils may have anti-inflammatory properties. Myristicin has been studied and shown that it inhibits the expression of cyclooxygenase-2 (COX-2).

Eating parsley regularly is also thought to speed up the excretion of uric acid. Uric acid can increase join stiffness and pain for those who suffer from arthritis, so this action means parsley can help reduce pain.

This "monster" of a juice recipe garners a lot of nutrients from all of the green foods on its ingredient list and is worth adding to your routine.

Per Serving
Calories: 74 | Fat: 0.5 g | Protein: 1.7 g | Sodium: 45 mg
Fiber: 0.0 g | Carbohydrates: 17.3 g | Sugar: 10.1 g

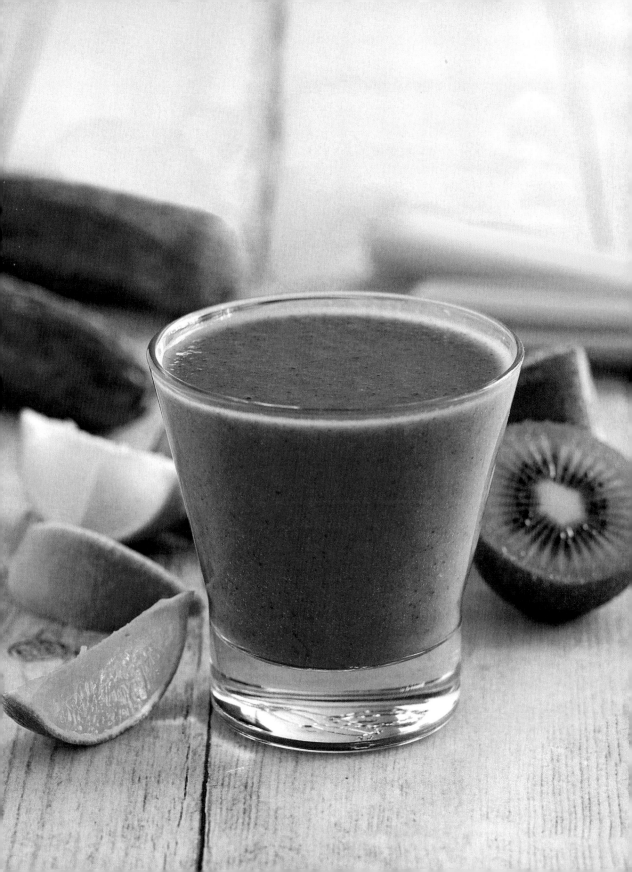

BEET CITY

Serves 1

INGREDIENTS

2 small beets
3 medium carrots
1 stalk celery
1 medium lemon, peeled and
    segmented

---

1 Prepare the beets by peeling and cutting them into appropriate-sized pieces for your juicer.

2 Prepare the carrots by removing the tops and tips and cutting them into appropriate-sized pieces for your juicer.

3 Prepare the celery stalk by removing the ends and cutting it into appropriate-sized pieces for your juicer.

4 Process the beets, carrots, celery, and lemon through the juicer.

5 Strain through a fine-mesh sieve if desired.

6 Consume immediately over ice or allow to chill in the refrigerator before serving.

7 Can be stored in a glass airtight container in the refrigerator up to 12 hours if using a centrifugal juicer and up to 3 days if using a masticating juicer.

KEY INGREDIENT: Beets

Beets are a unique source of betaine, known for its anti-inflammatory properties. Its anti-inflammatory action seems to come, in part, from its ability to interfere with pro-inflammatory signaling cascades. Betaine has also been shown to suppress pro-inflammatory cyclooxygenase-2 (COX-2). Interesting to note is that betaines target cell-signaling pathways at the molecular level, which means they have a similar mode of action to selective COX-2 inhibitor drugs such as aspirin and ibuprofen. Food is truly medicine in this case!

Raw beets are shown to retain betaine levels better than cooked beets, so juicing is an excellent option for getting the most nutrition from your beets. Beets are also a good source of folate, manganese, copper, and potassium.

Per Serving
Calories: 127 | Fat: 0.6 g | Protein: 1.3 g | Sodium: 286 mg
Fiber: 0.0 g | Carbohydrates: 27.8 g | Sugar: 21.8 g

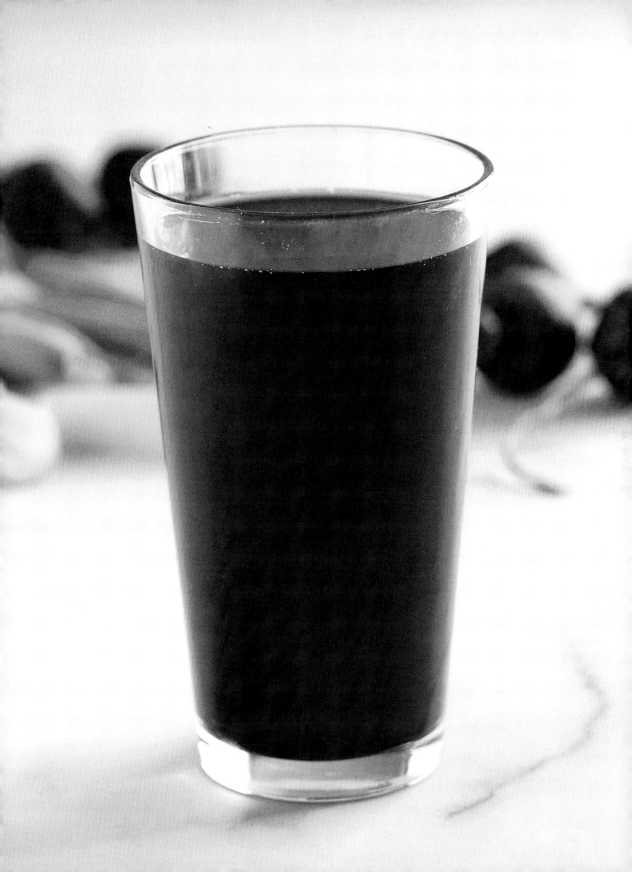

GREEN PAPAYA

Serves 2

INGREDIENTS

1 medium-large papaya
1 medium romaine heart

1 Prepare the papaya by peeling, removing seeds, and cutting it into appropriate-sized pieces for your juicer.

2 Prepare the romaine heart by removing the core and cutting it into appropriate-sized pieces for your juicer.

3 Process the papaya and romaine through the juicer.

4 Strain through a fine-mesh sieve if desired.

5 Consume immediately over ice or allow to chill in the refrigerator before serving.

6 Can be stored in a glass airtight container in the refrigerator up to 12 hours if using a centrifugal juicer and up to 3 days if using a masticating juicer.

KEY INGREDIENT: Papaya

Papaya contains a protein-digesting enzyme, papain. Papain (and other proteolytic enzymes, like the bromelain found in pineapple) modulates the inflammatory process in the body. It has been shown to reduce the swelling of mucous membranes and reduce capillary permeability. Papain increases the production of immune cells that speed healing. Papain also stimulates the digestion of proteins and fats and helps improve nutrient absorption.

In addition to anti-inflammatory papain, papaya is an excellent source of vitamins A and C. It's a good source of fiber, folate, magnesium, potassium, vitamin K, and copper as well. The potent antioxidants in papaya also contribute to its inflammation-fighting abilities.

This tropical fruit makes a lovely juice that pairs well with greens.

Per Serving
Calories: 156 | Fat: 0.9 g | Protein: 1.4 g | Sodium: 34 mg
Fiber: 0.0 g | Carbohydrates: 36.2 g | Sugar: 31.1 g

SWEET BABY RADICCHIO

Serves 1

INGREDIENTS

3 baby radicchio leaves
2 medium carrots
2 cups pineapple chunks (about ½ medium pineapple)

1 Prepare the radicchio leaves by chopping them into appropriate-sized pieces for your juicer.

2 Prepare the carrots by removing the tops and tips and cutting them into appropriate-sized pieces for your juicer.

3 Process the radicchio leaves, carrots, and pineapple chunks through your juicer.

4 Strain through a fine-mesh sieve if desired.

5 Consume immediately over ice or allow to chill in the refrigerator before serving.

6 Can be stored in a glass airtight container in the refrigerator up to 12 hours if using a centrifugal juicer and up to 3 days if using a masticating juicer.

KEY INGREDIENT: Radicchio

Radicchio, like most leafy vegetables, is rich in a number of key nutrients that help fight inflammation. Its bright red leaves indicate the presence of certain phytonutrients, one of which is ellagic acid. Ellagic acid is shown to block pro-inflammatory signaling pathways, in turn decreasing chronic inflammation. Radicchio also contains quercetin. Quercetin is a powerful flavonoid that inhibits production of inflammation-producing enzymes.

Radicchio also contains inulin, which helps support the body in many ways. Inulin promotes the discharge of pancreatic juices, indicating it can help aid digestion. Inulin is also a substance that can help regulate blood sugar levels.

Carrots and pineapple add to the nutrient level of this juice and also contribute to its sweetness since radicchio is not a naturally sweet vegetable.

Per Serving
Calories: 196 | Fat: 0.4 g | Protein: 1.3 g | Sodium: 92 mg
Fiber: 0.0 g | Carbohydrates: 47.8 g | Sugar: 38.4 g

Chapter 4
COLD DRINKS

What are you drinking on a daily basis? There's no reason why you can't make all of your everyday drinks inflammation-fighting drinks! The cold drinks in this chapter consist of the refreshments you probably already consume on a regular basis: milk, iced tea, lemonade, and even alternatives to sodas and sports drinks. In this chapter you'll find a number of nondairy milk recipes. Dairy is thought to cause inflammation, and it's easy to use alternatives that taste great and are often lower calorie than cow's milk. All of the drinks in this chapter are lower in sugar than most mainstream drinks you may be accustomed to and are all naturally sweetened or unsweetened. The last thing you want to do is counteract the anti-inflammatory ingredients you're utilizing with refined sugar! These recipes will help you replace your everyday drinks with inflammation-fighting drinks.

BASIC UNSWEETENED ALMOND MILK

Serves 4

INGREDIENTS

½ cup raw, whole, unsalted almonds
6 cups filtered water, divided

---

1 Cover the almonds with 2 cups filtered water in a small bowl and allow to soak at least 8 hours.

2 Use a fine-mesh strainer to drain and rinse the almonds.

3 Place the almonds in a large blender and add 4 cups filtered water to the blender.

4 Blend on high until smooth.

5 Strain the milk through a nut milk bag or cheesecloth.

6 Transfer to an airtight container and store in the refrigerator up to 5 days.

KEY INGREDIENT: Almonds

This recipe for unsweetened almond milk does double duty: it helps you eliminate inflammatory cow's milk from your diet while also using an ingredient that helps you fight inflammation. Smart!

Almonds are full of healthy polyunsaturated and monounsaturated fats, and they are also a great source of vitamin E. Not only are almonds thought to be anti-inflammatory, but they are a nutrient-dense food that has also been shown to help lower cholesterol. The almond milk you buy in the store if often filled with unnecessary ingredients, so making your own at home is a fantastic way to control what's going into your body. This recipe is economical, as it uses the least amount of almonds needed to create a milk. It's best for using in cooking or baking but not necessarily for drinking alone since it's not as creamy or flavorful as other milks.

Per Serving
Calories: 70 | Fat: 7.0 g | Protein: 3.0 g | Sodium: 0 mg
Fiber: 0.0 g | Carbohydrates: 1.5 g | Sugar: 0.5 g

ICED MOCHA LATTE

Serves 1

INGREDIENTS

1 cup cold coffee
1 tablespoon coconut oil
1 tablespoon full-fat canned coconut
  milk
2 teaspoons erythritol
1 tablespoon raw cacao powder
Ice, as needed

1 Place all ingredients, except
   ice, in a small blender.

2 Blend on high until thoroughly
   combined and frothy.

3 Fill a glass with ice and pour
   the latte over ice to consume
   immediately or store in an airtight container in the refrigerator up to 2 days.

KEY INGREDIENT: Raw Cacao Powder

In addition to raw cacao powder being an antioxidant power-house that fights inflammation, it is packed with a number of nutrients that provide health benefits.

The most common nutritional deficiency worldwide is iron deficiency. One of the great benefits of consuming raw cacao powder is that it's the most abundant source of plant-based iron. This is especially beneficial for vegans and vegetarians who don't consume animal products. Raw cacao powder is also one of the richest plant-based sources of magnesium, which happens to be another one of the most common nutritional deficiencies in the world. Magnesium is an important nutrient for both brain and heart health.

As you can see raw cacao powder is a great choice for fighting inflammation and delivering key nutrients to your body!

Per Serving
Calories: 168 | Fat: 16.3 g | Protein: 1.6 g | Sodium: 5 mg
Fiber: 1.0 g | Carbohydrates: 11.4 g | Sugar: 0.0 g

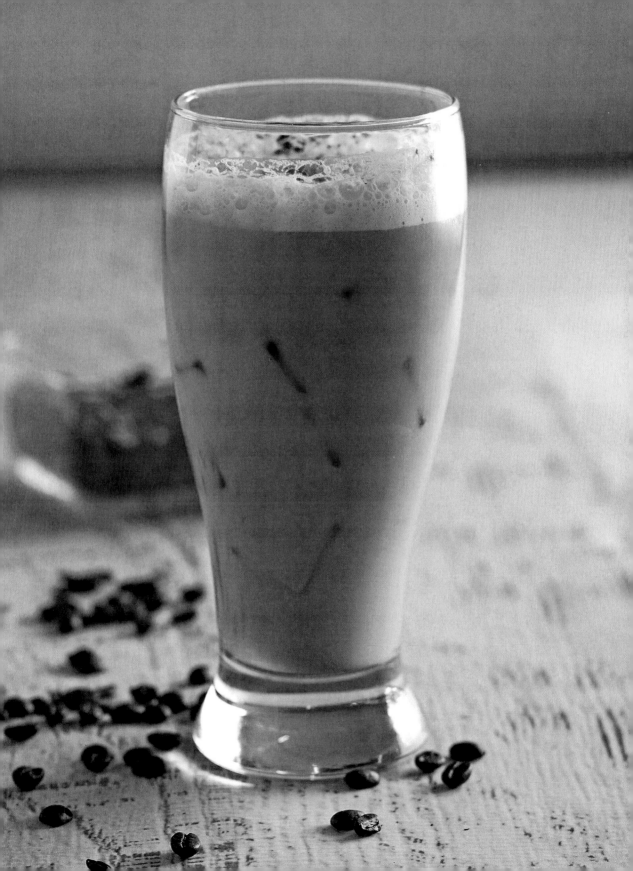

CREAMY VANILLA WALNUT MILK

Serves 4

INGREDIENTS

1 cup walnut pieces
6 cups filtered water, divided
1 teaspoon pure vanilla extract
1 tablespoon pure maple syrup

1 Cover the walnuts with 2 cups filtered water and soak at least 8 hours.

2 Use a fine-mesh strainer to drain and rinse the walnuts.

3 Place the walnuts in a large blender, along with 4 cups filtered water, vanilla extract, and maple syrup.

4 Blend on high until smooth.

5 Strain the milk through a nut milk bag or cheesecloth.

6 Transfer to an airtight container and store in the refrigerator up to 5 days.

KEY INGREDIENT: Walnuts

Walnuts are a smart choice for a dairy milk alternative. They have an excellent nutritional profile, and using them as milk is a great way to include them in your diet. In fact, of all the nuts, walnuts are the richest source of omega-3 fatty acids. Walnuts are also a good source of vitamin E, which is important for immune system function. These powerful nuts have been well studied for their protective benefits to the heart and circulatory system.

Walnuts have a number of elements that are known to fight inflammation, including alpha-linolenic fatty acid, the amino acid L-arginine, and phenolic antioxidants. Researchers have found that walnuts inhibit the production of the neurotransmitter substance P and bradykinin, which increase pain and inflammation in the body. The anti-inflammatory nutrients found in walnuts are also thought to have anticancer benefits.

Per Serving
Calories: 204 | Fat: 18.7 g | Protein: 4.6 g | Sodium: 1 mg
Fiber: 0.0 g | Carbohydrates: 5.6 g | Sugar: 3.9 g

CREAMY VANILLA ALMOND MILK

Serves 4

INGREDIENTS

1 cup whole almonds
5 cups filtered water, divided
1 teaspoon pure vanilla extract
1 tablespoon pure maple syrup

---

1 Cover the almonds in a small bowl with 2 cups filtered water and allow to soak at least 8 hours.

2 Use a fine-mesh strainer to drain and rinse the almonds.

3 Place the almonds in a large blender, along with 3 cups filtered water, vanilla extract, and maple syrup.

4 Blend on high until smooth.

5 Strain the milk through a nut milk bag or cheesecloth.

6 Transfer to an airtight container and store in the refrigerator up to 5 days.

KEY INGREDIENT: Almonds

The regular consumption of almonds has been shown to lower C-reactive protein levels, a key marker of inflammation and an independent risk factor for heart disease. Almonds may also be cardioprotective because they reduce the inflammation of blood vessels and for their ability to help lower LDL cholesterol levels. In addition, almonds contain the compound salicin. Salicin is a natural anti-inflammatory agent that converts to salicylic acid inside the body. This is the same active ingredient in aspirin!

Almonds are also high in vitamin E, which is shown to nourish and have an antiaging effect on your skin. The type of vitamin E found in almonds is known to be a powerful antioxidant that fights free radical damage and oxidative stress.

This Creamy Vanilla Almond Milk is a creamier, thicker almond milk than the basic version found earlier in this chapter. It's great for drinking or when you want more almond flavor.

Per Serving
Calories: 202 | Fat: 17.0 g | Protein: 7.6 g | Sodium: 0 mg
Fiber: 0.0 g | Carbohydrates: 6.7 g | Sugar: 4.7 g

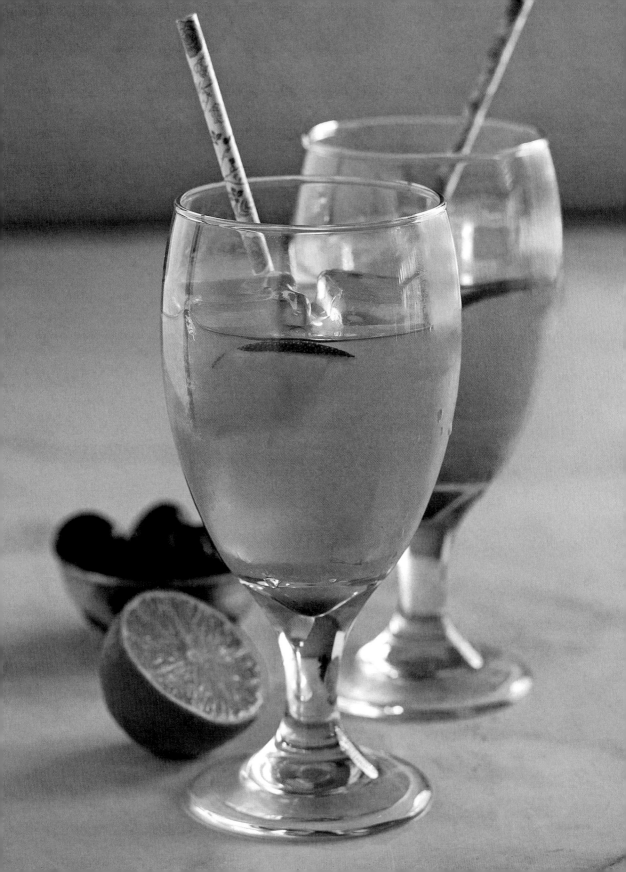

CHERRY LIMEADE

Serves 6

INGREDIENTS

4¾ cups water, divided
¾ cup fresh lime juice (from about 4 large limes)
2 cups pitted sweet cherries
½ cup erythritol

---

1 Combine 4½ cups water with the lime juice in a medium pitcher.

2 In a small saucepan, bring the cherries, erythritol, and ¼ cup water to a simmer over low heat.

3 Allow the cherry mixture to simmer, stirring occasionally, for 5 minutes.

4 Remove the cherry mixture from the heat and allow to cool.

5 Place the cherry mixture in a small blender and blend on high until you have a smooth purée.

6 Transfer the cherry purée to the pitcher and stir until it is combined with the limeade.

7 Allow to chill in the refrigerator before serving.

8 Serve over ice. May be stored in the refrigerator up to 4 days.

KEY INGREDIENT: Cherries

Cherries have a lower glycemic index than most fruits and are packed with nutrients. Their deep crimson hue indicates that they have an abundant amount of antioxidants and that they are rich in one type of antioxidant in particular: anthocyanins. Consumption of foods with high concentrations of anthocyanins is linked to decreased risk of several chronic inflammatory diseases, including cardiovascular disease, diabetes, and cancer.

Fresh or frozen cherries can be used for this drink. Frozen may be preferred for convenience since they are already pitted. If frozen are used, no changes to the recipe are necessary. The cherries give this limeade its bright pink color naturally and provide terrific flavor. Lemons can easily be substituted for the limes to make this cherry lemonade.

Per Serving
Calories: 39 | Fat: 0.1 g | Protein: 0.7 g | Sodium: 0 mg
Fiber: 1.2 g | Carbohydrates: 26.8 g | Sugar: 7.1 g
Sugar Alcohol: 16.0 g

UNSWEETENED RASPBERRY ICED TEA

Serves 4

INGREDIENTS

4 cups plus 2 tablespoons water, divided
4 green tea bags
6 ounces fresh raspberries
Ice, as needed

---

1   Place 4 cups water and 4 tea bags in a glass airtight container and place in the refrigerator.

2   Let the tea cold brew for 5 hours in the refrigerator.

3   Meanwhile, heat the fresh raspberries with 2 tablespoons of water in a small saucepan over medium heat.

4   Allow the raspberries to simmer until they are completely broken down, about 5 minutes.

5   Remove from heat and use a fine-mesh strainer to remove the seeds.

6   After 5 hours, remove the tea bags from the water. Combine the tea and raspberry purée.

7   Serve over ice. May be stored in the refrigerator up to 4 days.

KEY INGREDIENT: Raspberries

Those who are interested in anti-inflammatory foods for their antiaging effects will want to consume raspberries frequently. Raspberries contain ellagic acid, a polyphenol compound present in a lot of berries, but at the highest levels in raspberries. Ellagic acid is just one of the anti-inflammatory phytonutrients found in raspberries, and studies have found that it prevents collagen degradation by blocking matrix metalloproteinase production. In addition, it diminishes the production of pro-inflammatory cytokines. That means it helps prevent wrinkles and skin issues caused by inflammation!

Ellagic acid does more, however, than just combat aging. It's been shown to help prevent overactivity and overproduction of a number of pro-inflammatory enzymes, which can have a positive effect on inflammation in the body. For example, ellagic acid seems to help with excessive inflammation associated with Crohn's disease.

In addition to ellagic acid, raspberries are an excellent source of vitamin C, manganese, and fiber. They also have a good amount of B vitamins, folic acid, copper, and iron. The raspberries make this unsweetened tea an inviting, bright pink color and add just a touch of flavor.

Per Serving
Calories: 24 | Fat: 0.2 g | Protein: 0.5 g | Sodium: 0 mg
Fiber: 2.8 g | Carbohydrates: 5.8 g | Sugar: 1.9 g

BETTER SWEET TEA

Serves 8

INGREDIENTS

8 cups water
8 green tea bags
¼ cup erythritol
Ice, as needed

---

1 Place 8 cups water and 8 tea bags in a glass airtight container and place in the refrigerator.

2 Let the tea cold brew in the refrigerator for 5 hours.

3 After 5 hours, remove the tea bags from the tea.

4 Add erythritol and stir until dissolved.

5 Serve over ice. May be stored in the refrigerator up to 4 days.

KEY INGREDIENT: Green Tea

Green tea has a long history in China and very early on was ingrained as a fundamental part of Chinese society. Today it's used by traditional Chinese medicine practitioners to reduce heat, relieve headaches, aid digestion, and offer other health benefits. Green tea is loaded with antioxidants, like many of the inflammation-reducing foods highlighted in this book. It has two especially impressive compounds that help it fight inflammation: epigallocatechin gallate (EGCG) and quercetin. In studies, EGCG has been shown to reduce inflammation markers. Quercetin fights inflammation by suppressing inflammation pathways and functions. This is why green tea is a great choice when making iced tea.

Instead of sweetening this Better Sweet Tea with refined white sugar, which can cause inflammation, erythritol is used. Erythritol is a natural sugar alcohol that is found in plants. It does not induce an insulin response or change glucose metabolism in the body. This makes it a smart choice for sweetening your tea. It can be found in the natural section of most well-stocked grocery stores.

Per Serving

Calories: 2 | Fat: 0.0 g | Protein: 0.0 g | Sodium: 0 mg
Fiber: 0.0 g | Carbohydrates: 6.7 g | Sugar: 0.0 g
Sugar Alcohol: 6.0 g

BLUEBERRY LEMONADE

Serves 6
INGREDIENTS

4¾ cups water, divided
1 cup fresh-squeezed lemon juice
(from 4–5 large lemons)
2 cups blueberries
½ cup erythritol
Ice, as needed

1 In a large pitcher, mix together 4½ cups water with lemon juice.

2 Heat the blueberries, ¼ cup water, and erythritol in a small saucepan over medium heat.

3 Bring the blueberry mixture to a simmer and allow to simmer 5 minutes.

4 Remove the blueberry mixture from the heat and allow to cool.

5 In a large blender, blend the blueberry mixture on high until you have a smooth purée.

6 Add the blueberry purée to the lemonade and stir until well combined. Strain if desired.

7 Serve over ice. May be stored in the refrigerator up to 4 days.

KEY INGREDIENT: Lemon

Lemons are often used for flavoring in cooking, but many people overlook their tremendous health-promoting properties. Lemons feature phytonutrients with antioxidant and antibiotic effects and are an excellent source of vitamin C.

Lemons contain beta-cryptoxanthin, which belongs to a class of carotenoids. Beta-cryptoxanthin is a strong antioxidant that prevents free radical damage. It is thought that this helps it protect against the oxidative damage that can result in inflammation. One population-based, prospective study computed the dietary carotenoid intakes of subjects using diet diaries. It was found that a modest increase in beta-cryptoxanthin, such as is found in one glass of orange juice, significantly lowered one's risk of developing inflammatory disorders such as rheumatoid arthritis by 40 percent. This presents a strong case for drinking healthy lemonade!

Store-bought lemonade is made with loads of refined sugar and often doesn't even use real lemon juice. Skip the grocery store stuff and make it at home without refined sugar! It's so much easier than most people assume, and you'll reap the health benefits.

Per Serving
Calories: 36 | Fat: 0.1 g | Protein: 0.5 g | Sodium: 0 mg
Fiber: 1.3 g | Carbohydrates: 26.0 g | Sugar: 5.9 g
Sugar Alcohol: 16.0 g

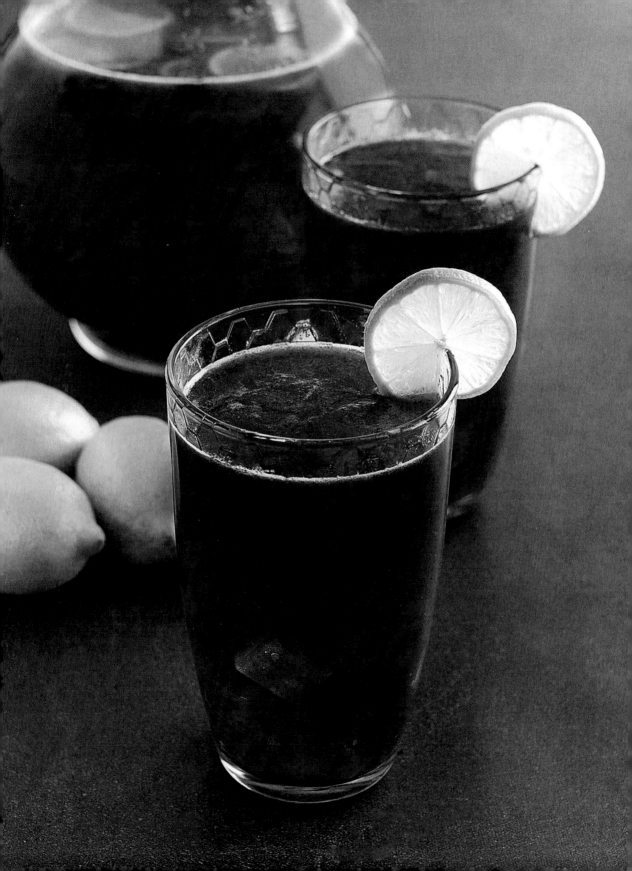

BLUEBERRY SWEET TEA

Serves 8

INGREDIENTS

8 cups plus 2 tablespoons water, divided
8 green tea bags
1 cup blueberries
¼ cup erythritol
Ice, as needed

1 Place 8 cups water and 8 tea bags in a glass airtight container and place in the refrigerator.

2 Let the tea cold brew in the refrigerator for 5 hours.

3 Meanwhile, in a small saucepan, heat the blueberries, 2 tablespoons water, and erythritol over medium heat.

4 Bring the blueberry mixture to a simmer and allow to simmer 5 minutes. Remove from heat and allow to cool.

5 In a large blender, blend the blueberry mixture on high until you have a smooth purée.

6 After 5 hours, remove the tea bags from the tea.

7 Add the blueberry purée to the tea and stir until well combined. Strain if desired.

8 Serve over ice. May be stored in the refrigerator up to 4 days.

KEY INGREDIENT: Blueberries

Blueberries give this sweet tea a powerful upgrade! They are deeply pigmented and have a unique combination of phytonutrients. Blueberries have a wide range of flavonoids that give them a host of health benefits. While they are best known for their anthocyanin flavonoids, they also have two other unique anti-inflammatory phytonutrients, resveratrol and pterostilbene. Both of these belong to the group of compounds known as *stilbenoids*. These two powerful phytonutrients have been studied for their effects on pathways in inflammatory conditions and were found to down-regulate Akt phosphorylation (a well-known marker for inflammatory conditions). Pterostilbene was also found to suppress inflammatory edema and down-regulate inflammatory mediators.

Nature is a beautiful thing because these wonderful properties also contribute to the incredible flavor in blueberries. In addition to their health benefits, blueberries improve the taste of your beverages, like this Blueberry Sweet Tea!

Per Serving

Calories: 12 | Fat: 0.1 g | Protein: 0.1 g | Sodium: 0 mg
Fiber: 0.4 g | Carbohydrates: 9.4 g | Sugar: 1.8 g
Sugar Alcohol: 6.0 g

MACA CHOCOLATE MILK

Serves 4

INGREDIENTS

4 cups unsweetened vanilla almond milk
8 pitted dates
½ cup raw cacao powder
1 tablespoon maca root powder
¼ teaspoon pure stevia powder

---

1 Place all ingredients in a large blender.

2 Blend on high until the dates are thoroughly combined and the mixture is completely smooth, 1–2 minutes.

3 Chill before serving. May be stored in an airtight container in the refrigerator up to 5 days.

KEY INGREDIENT: Maca Root

Maca is a starchy root vegetable that is grown in South America. You won't find it served at restaurants or even in your grocery store, though. Thankfully, this superfood is found in powder form in most health food stores and is readily available online. Maca root was first used by the Incas over 2,000 years ago. They relied on it for its ability to give them sustained energy and endurance. It's easy to see why it was so important to the Incas when you discover that the maca root has more than fifty-five different beneficial phytochemicals.

Maca root has many medicinal purposes. It's been shown to enhance your memory and your mood and give your immune system a boost. It's used for its antiaging properties as well as treating adrenal fatigue. One way it's thought to help with inflammation is by regulating inflammatory hormones like cortisol. Maca has also been found to reduce inflammation at the cellular level.

This Maca Chocolate Milk is rich and creamy and tastes much more indulgent than it is!

Per Serving
Calories: 125 | Fat: 4.0 g | Protein: 4.1 g | Sodium: 180 mg
Fiber: 4.9 g | Carbohydrates: 21.7 g | Sugar: 10.2 g

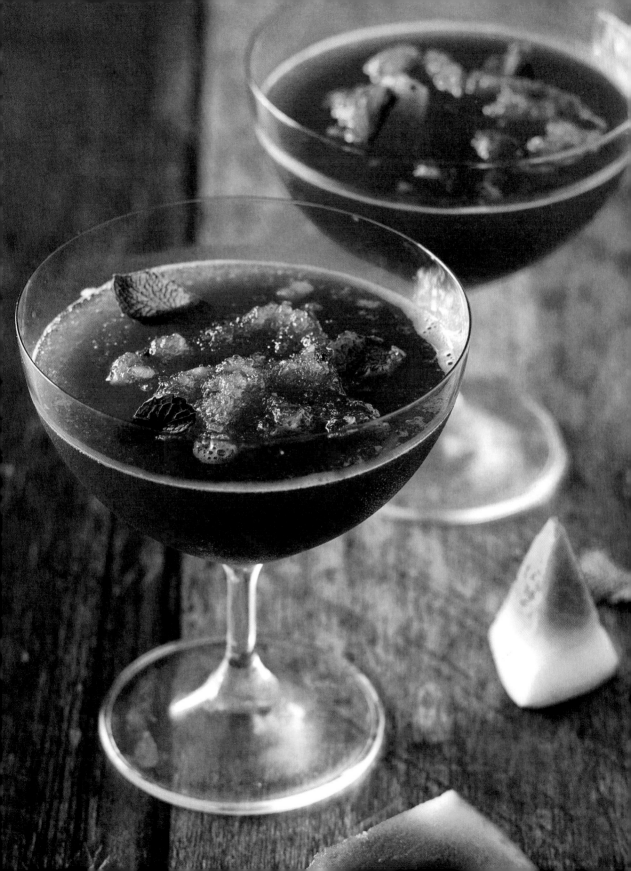

WATERMELON MINT MOCKTAIL

Serves 2

INGREDIENTS

2 cups cubed watermelon
1 tablespoon raw honey
6 whole mint leaves
Ice, as needed
½ cup sparkling water

1   Place the watermelon cubes and honey in a large blender.

2   Blend the watermelon and honey on high until you have a smooth liquid.

3   Place the mint leaves in the bottom of a cocktail shaker. Use a muddler to muddle the mint leaves until they are just broken down slightly.

4   Fill the cocktail shaker with ice.

5   Add the watermelon mixture to the cocktail shaker and add a lid. Shake the cocktail shaker vigorously for 20 seconds.

6   Fill two glasses with ice. Strain the contents of the cocktail shaker evenly into the two glasses.

7   Top each glass with ¼ cup sparkling water.

8   Consume immediately.

KEY INGREDIENT: Watermelon

Nothing says summer like watermelon. Even though watermelon is 92 percent water, it still contains plenty of nutrients. Watermelon provides good amounts of vitamins C, A, and B_6. The anti-inflammatory benefits from watermelon come from a number of phytonutrients, with the standout being lycopene. Watermelons have one of the highest levels of lycopene among all fruits and vegetables. In fact, watermelons have a higher concentration of lycopene than red tomatoes, which are famous for their lycopene content. The lycopene in watermelons is also highly bioavailable. Lycopene is significant because it suppresses various pro-inflammatory cytokines. Be sure to give the watermelon a chance to ripen. Using ripe watermelon is important; the redder the fruit, the more lycopene it contains.

This is a refreshing drink that takes full advantage of watermelon's natural sweetness. Instead of a cocktail, why not fight inflammation with this mocktail?

Per Serving
Calories: 77 | Fat: 0.4 g | Protein: 1.0 g | Sodium: 1 mg
Fiber: 0.7 g | Carbohydrates: 20.3 g | Sugar: 18.1 g

MANGO LIME FIZZ

Serves 2

INGREDIENTS

1 medium mango
1 cup water
2 tablespoons lime juice
Ice, as needed
½ cup club soda

1   Peel the mango, remove the core, and cut the mango into chunks.

2   Place the mango chunks, water, and lime juice into a large blender.

3   Blend on high until the ingredients are thoroughly combined and smooth.

4   Fill two medium glasses with ice.

5   Pour the mango mixture over the ice. Add ¼ cup club soda to each glass and stir.

6   Consume immediately.

KEY INGREDIENT: Mango

Mango is a sweet, luscious fruit grown mostly in the tropics that is high in many nutrients. Luckily, it's available year-round in grocery stores. Mangoes are a great source of vitamin C, B vitamins, fiber, and copper. Mangoes have been shown to help lower blood glucose levels and help manage high blood pressure. Mango is high in vitamin B_6, which makes it a great food for a healthy brain, as vitamin B_6 and other B vitamins are crucial for maintaining healthy neurotransmitters. As for its anti-inflammatory effects, one study showed that consuming mango led to decreased intestinal inflammation and levels of pro-inflammatory cytokines.

This Mango Lime Fizz makes a refreshing, delicious, and healthy soda alternative for those who crave carbonation in their drinks.

Per Serving
Calories: 104 | Fat: 0.5 g | Protein: 1.4 g | Sodium: 13 mg
Fiber: 2.8 g | Carbohydrates: 26.4 g | Sugar: 23.2 g

COCONUT LIME SPORTS DRINK

Serves 4

INGREDIENTS

3 cups unsweetened coconut water
1 cup water
½ cup fresh lime juice
¼ teaspoon sea salt
½ teaspoon pure stevia powder

1 In a medium container, combine the coconut water, water, and lime juice.

2 Add the sea salt and stevia powder and stir until dissolved.

3 Consume immediately or store in an airtight container up to 1 week.

KEY INGREDIENT: Coconut Water

Coconut water is a naturally hydrating drink that can help replace electrolytes lost during rigorous exercise. Electrolytes are important minerals that play crucial roles in your body, including maintaining proper fluid balance.

Research has shown that both young and mature coconut water has anti-inflammatory properties. In one study, coconut water was found to have the same ability as ibuprofen to suppress inflammatory responses in the body. Researchers haven't concluded what the exact mode of action is, but the results of lowered inflammation in the body were clear.

With no added sugars or artificial flavors or colors, this sports drink is a much smarter option for hydrating.

Per Serving
Calories: 41 | Fat: 0.4 g | Protein: 1.4 g | Sodium: 287 mg
Fiber: 2.1 g | Carbohydrates: 9.3 g | Sugar: 5.0 g

UNSWEETENED ICED CINNAMON COFFEE

Serves 1

INGREDIENTS

1 cup brewed coffee
¼ teaspoon ground cinnamon
¼ teaspoon pure vanilla extract
1 tablespoon full-fat coconut milk
Ice, as needed

1 Place all ingredients, except ice, in a small blender.

2 Blend on high until the ingredients are thoroughly combined.

3 Fill a glass with ice. Pour the coffee mixture over ice.

4 Consume immediately.

KEY INGREDIENT: Cinnamon

Cinnamon is one of the most delicious spices and is used frequently in baking to add a warm depth to coffee cakes, crisps, and more. Not only does cinnamon have a lovely flavor, but it also comes with a host of health benefits. Cinnamon has been used for its medicinal properties for centuries. It is considered antimicrobial, antifungal, and antidiabetic and is known to help control blood sugar levels. Cinnamon gets its anti-inflammatory fighting powers from two powerful compounds, E-cinnamaldehyde and O-methoxycinnamaldehyde. Both of these compounds have been shown to decrease chronic inflammation through the down-regulation of nitric oxide and TNF-α production.

Cinnamon is especially high in antioxidants, which help fight inflammation caused by oxidative stress. In fact, it ranks seventh for antioxidants of all foods, spices, and herbs on the Oxygen Radical Absorbance Capacity (ORAC) scale.

Per Serving
Calories: 35 | Fat: 3.0 g | Protein: 0.6 g | Sodium: 5 mg
Fiber: 0.4 g | Carbohydrates: 1.1 g | Sugar: 0.2 g

STRAWBERRY SAGE LEMONADE

Serves 6

INGREDIENTS

1 cup lemon juice (from 4–5 large
    lemons)
4¼ cups water, divided
1 pound strawberries, hulled and cut
    in half
1 cup sage leaves
½ cup erythritol
Ice, as needed

---

1 In a large pitcher, combine the
     lemon juice with 4 cups water.

2 In a medium saucepan, heat
     the strawberries, sage leaves,
     erythritol, and ¼ cup water
     over medium heat and bring
     to a boil.

3 Once the mixture is boiling, use
     the back of a wooden spoon
     or a potato masher to mash
     the strawberries.

4 Reduce the heat and let the
     mixture simmer 3–4 minutes.
     Remove from heat and allow
     to cool.

5 Transfer the strawberry mixture
     to a large blender. Blend the
     strawberry mixture on high until
     the strawberries and sage are
     thoroughly combined and you
     have a smooth purée.

6 Pour the purée into the lemon-
     ade and stir well.

7 Serve over ice. May be stored
     in the refrigerator up to 4 days.

KEY INGREDIENT: Sage

Many herbs have been used for holistic remedies for centuries. Sage has some powerful compounds in its leaves that contribute to the anti-inflammatory effect it has. Carnosic acid and carnosol are the main anti-inflammatory compounds present in sage and its sister herb, rosemary. These compounds have both antioxidant and antimicrobial properties. Studies have shown that these compounds target multiple pathways associated with inflammation and cancer.

Sage also contains several antioxidant enzymes, including superoxide dismutase (SOD) and peroxide, and rosmarinic acid, which is a potent anti-inflammatory agent. Rosmarinic acid is readily absorbed by the body and is often recommended for patients with inflammatory conditions like RA and atherosclerosis.

Sage adds a unique and sophisticated flavor to this lemonade recipe. It pairs very well with strawberries, which of course also add to the anti-inflammatory abilities of this drink.

Per Serving
Calories: 33 | Fat: 0.2 g | Protein: 0.8 g | Sodium: 2 mg
Fiber: 1.8 g | Carbohydrates: 24.6 g | Sugar: 4.3 g
Sugar Alcohol: 16.0 g

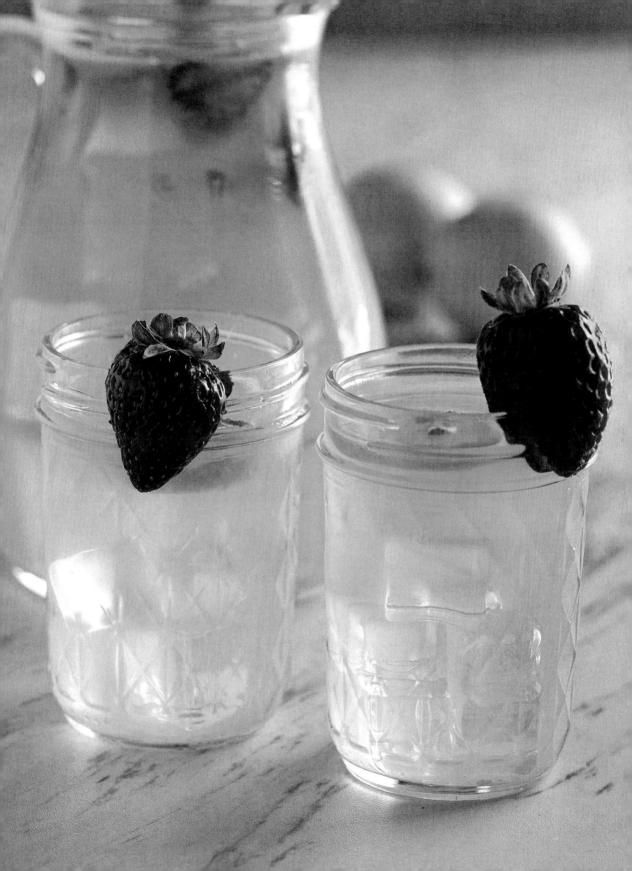

ROSEMARY COCONUT COOLER

Serves 1

INGREDIENTS

1 cup unsweetened coconut water
1 tablespoon rosemary leaves
¼ teaspoon pure stevia powder
Ice, as needed
1 cup club soda

1 Combine the coconut water, rosemary leaves, and stevia powder in a small blender.

2 Blend on high until the ingredients are thoroughly combined.

3 Pour the coconut water mixture over a tall glass of ice. Add the club soda and stir.

4 Consume immediately.

KEY INGREDIENT: Rosemary

Rosemary has similar inflammation-fighting compounds to sage. Two of the compounds found in rosemary that fight inflammation are apigenin and diosmin. These two compounds have an anti-inflammatory effect through their ability to prevent your body from producing prostaglandins, which are responsible for causing an inflammation reaction throughout your body. The compound rosmarinic acid present in rosemary also fights inflammation in this way.

Rosemary is common in cooking but less common in drinks. Paired with coconut water, club soda, and a little stevia, this drink with inflammation-fighting rosemary makes a healthy alternative for anyone who enjoys soda. Its unique flavor is perfect for adult palates.

Per Serving
Calories: 47 | Fat: 0.6 g | Protein: 1.8 g | Sodium: 301 mg
Fiber: 2.8 g | Carbohydrates: 9.4 g | Sugar: 6.0 g

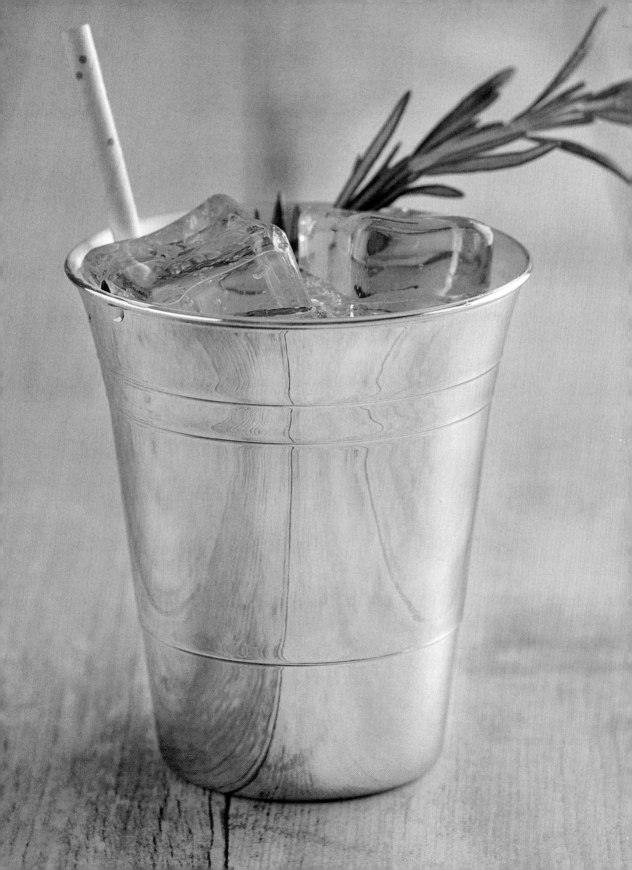

GINGER ALE

Serves 6
INGREDIENTS

For the Ginger Syrup
2 cups water
1½ cups peeled, chopped fresh
   ginger
½ cup pure maple syrup

For the Ginger Ale
4½ cups club soda
1½ cups Ginger Syrup

---

1 First, make the Ginger Syrup.
   Heat the water and ginger in a
   small saucepan over medium-
   low heat to a very low simmer.

2 Let the water simmer, with the
   pan partially covered, for 45
   minutes. Keep the simmer very
   low.

3 Remove from heat and cover.
   Let steep 20 minutes.

4 Strain the ginger through a
   fine-mesh sieve, pushing down
   on the ginger with the back of
   a wooden spoon to release all
   liquid.

5 Add maple syrup to the ginger
   mixture and stir to combine.
   Ginger Syrup may be kept in
   an airtight container in the
   refrigerator up to 1 week.

6 For each serving of Ginger Ale:
   pour ¾ cup club soda into a
   glass. Top with ¼ cup Ginger
   Syrup and stir to combine.

KEY INGREDIENT: Ginger

Ginger originated in Southeast Asia over 5,000 years ago and was considered a luxury. It was widely cultivated and traded in other countries. Ginger has been traded throughout the centuries and prized for its medicinal merits. It became a highly sought-after commodity in Europe. In the Middle Ages, just one pound of the coveted spice was worth as much as one sheep.

While for thousands of years ginger was purported to be used for the treatment of a variety of ailments, like many herbal remedies, much of the information was passed down by word of mouth and there wasn't always scientific evidence to back the claims. Today, however, ginger has been studied extensively for its medicinal properties and health benefits. It is widely accepted that there is ample scientific evidence and research to support ginger's role as an antioxidant, anti-inflammatory agent, anti-nausea compound, and anticancer agent, as well as the protective effect of ginger against a host of other diseases.

Per Serving
Calories: 70 | Fat: 0.0 g | Protein: 0.1 g | Sodium: 40 mg
Fiber: 0.1 g | Carbohydrates: 18.0 g | Sugar: 15.9 g

SPARKLING WATERMELON LIME DRINK

Serves 8

INGREDIENTS

5 cups watermelon cubes
½ cup fresh lime juice
5 cups unsweetened lime-flavored
  sparkling water

---

1 In a large blender, in batches if necessary, blend the watermelon cubes until they are completely smooth.

2 Transfer the watermelon juice to a large pitcher. Stir in the lime juice and sparkling water.

3 Allow to chill before serving. Serve over ice. May be stored in the refrigerator up to 4 days.

KEY INGREDIENT: Watermelon

Watermelon is such a hydrating fruit, so it makes a smart choice to include in drink recipes. It is high in potassium, making it a natural electrolyte that can help regulate the action of nerves and muscles in your body. Watermelon also has an alkaline-forming effect on the body, which can help counteract the effects of consuming too many high acid–producing foods, such as meat and dairy.

While the lycopene in watermelon is one compound responsible for the fruit's anti-inflammatory action, there are more at work. Another compound found in watermelons, Cucurbitacin E, also contributes to its ability to fight inflammation. Cucurbitacin E is an anti-inflammatory agent because it blocks pro-inflammatory cyclooxygenase enzymes.

Per Serving
Calories: 32 | Fat: 0.1 g | Protein: 0.6 g | Sodium: 1 mg
Fiber: 0.4 g | Carbohydrates: 8.5 g | Sugar: 6.2 g

ORANGE STRAWBERRY FIZZ

Serves 1

INGREDIENTS

4 large strawberries, hulled
1 tablespoon water
Ice, as needed
¾ cup fresh orange juice
¼ cup soda water

1 In a small blender, blend the strawberries and water on high until they form a smooth purée. Set aside.

2 Put the ice in a glass. Pour the orange juice in the glass and top it with the soda water.

3 Stir in the strawberry purée.

4 Consume immediately.

KEY INGREDIENT: Strawberries

Strawberries are among the most popular fruits consumed throughout the world. Not only are these berries scrumptious, but they are also highly nutritious and health-promoting. Strawberries score approximately a 40 on the glycemic index. This is a low number compared to many fresh fruits. Researchers have found that consumption of strawberries following a meal has a positive impact on the regulation of insulin and blood sugar levels. Strawberries contain a number of anti-inflammatory polyphenols, including ellagitannins. The ellagitannins in strawberries have been found to block inflammatory actions in the body.

This Orange Strawberry Fizz is another great soda alternative and is a beautifully colored drink.

Per Serving
Calories: 106 | Fat: 0.3 g | Protein: 1.8 g | Sodium: 13 mg
Fiber: 1.8 g | Carbohydrates: 24.9 g | Sugar: 19.1 g

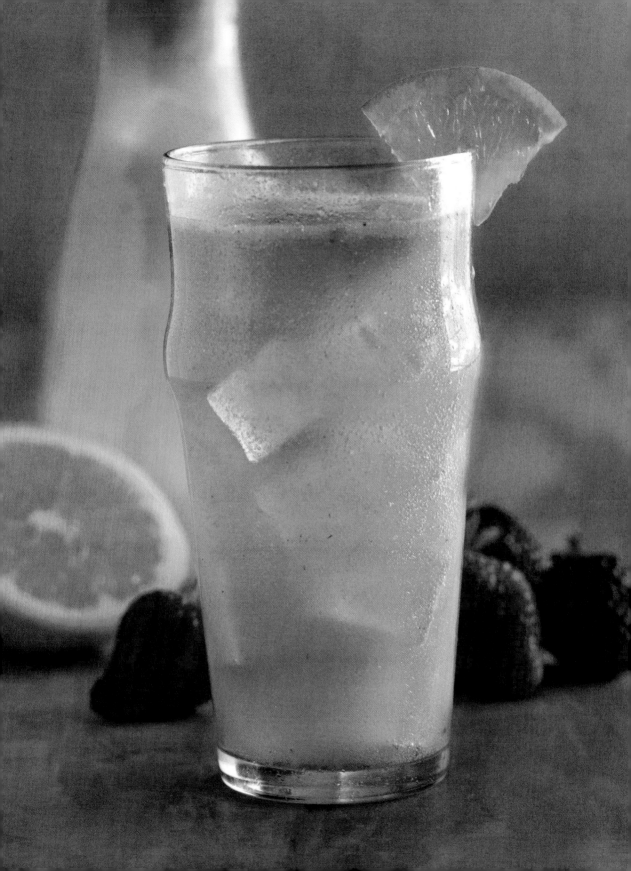

CHERRY SODA

Serves 4
INGREDIENTS

For the Cherry Syrup
1½ cups fresh pitted sweet cherries
1½ cups water
½ teaspoon pure stevia powder

For the Cherry Soda
3 cups club soda
1 cup Cherry Syrup

---

1 First, make the Cherry Syrup. Heat the cherries and water in a small saucepan over medium heat to a simmer. Allow to simmer 10 minutes.

2 While the cherries and water are simmering, mash the cherries to release more flavor.

3 Remove from heat and strain the cherries through a fine-mesh sieve. Use the back of a wooden spoon to remove as much liquid from the cherries as possible.

4 Stir in stevia. Cherry Syrup may be stored in an airtight container in the refrigerator up to 1 week.

5 For each serving of Cherry Soda: pour ¾ cup club soda into a glass. Top with ¼ cup Cherry Syrup and stir to combine.

KEY INGREDIENT: Sweet Cherries

There are different varieties of cherries, including sweet and tart cherries. Both sweet and tart cherries are known for their health-promoting properties. A number of human studies have been done researching the health benefits of cherries. The cumulative results of these studies show that cherries have been found to reduce oxidative stress in the body, decrease markers for inflammation, decrease muscle soreness after exercise, decrease blood pressure and arthritis symptoms, improve sleep, and decrease triglycerides and HDL ratios in obese patients. Polyphenols, melatonin, carotenoids, and vitamins E and C all contribute to the antioxidant and anti-inflammatory properties of cherries. All together, these nutrients form a powerful anti-inflammatory punch that can have a positive effect on many aspects of your health.

If you like to drink soda every day, this is an excellent replacement. Make a double or triple batch of the naturally sweetened Cherry Syrup to have on hand whenever a craving for soda hits.

Per Serving
Calories: 11 | Fat: 0.0 g | Protein: 0.2 g | Sodium: 37 mg
Fiber: 0.0 g | Carbohydrates: 2.7 g | Sugar: 2.5 g

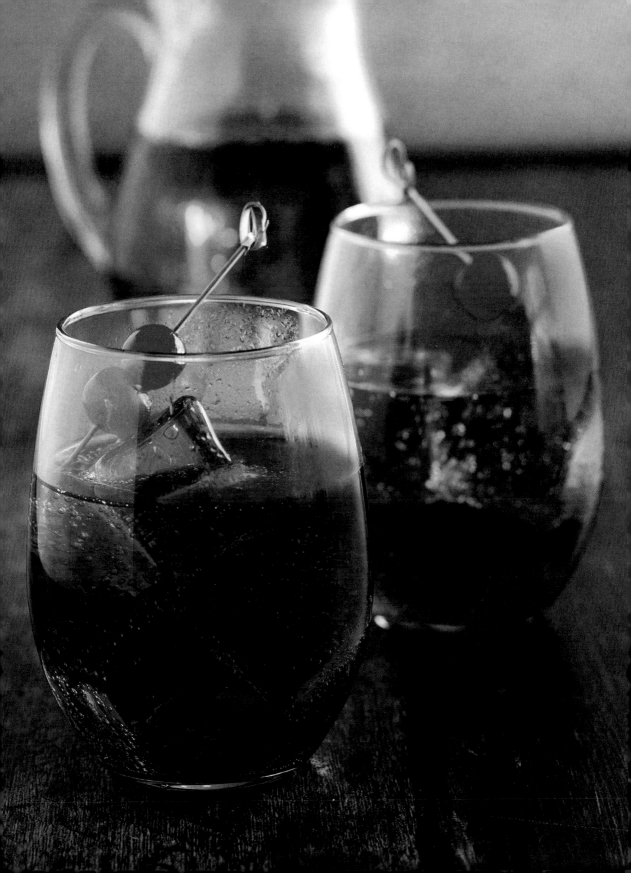

Chapter 5

TONICS AND SHOTS

While all the recipes in this book are designed to have anti-inflammatory effects through their ingredients, this chapter has recipes that were designed for specific ailments and needs. Tonics are drinks that can help you heal or feel better. Whether you are suffering from insomnia, digestive troubles, or a cold, there is likely a recipe in this chapter that is designed to help.

Fair warning: These recipes were not developed based on taste. Instead, they were designed specifically for their medicinal qualities. Some happen to taste great naturally, but all of the drinks, regardless of taste, have powerful healing ingredients that can help you if you're seeking natural solutions to whatever is ailing you.

The shot recipes can give you a quick anti-inflammatory boost. Like the tonics, many of them were designed for specific health concerns or to be used preventively. They are easy to consume quickly, and some of them may become part of your daily routine.

PASSION TONIC

Serves 1

INGREDIENTS

1 cup unsweetened pomegranate juice
1 teaspoon maca root powder

1 Pour the pomegranate juice into a glass.
2 Stir the maca root powder into the pomegranate juice until it is completely dissolved.
3 Consume immediately.

KEY INGREDIENT: Pomegranate

Pomegranates have become famous for their antioxidant abilities. That is thanks mostly to the powerful antioxidants found in their juice and peel called *punicalagins*. These punicalagins are such strong antioxidants that pomegranate juice has been found to have three times the antioxidant activity than that of red wine and green tea.

The effect of such a powerful antioxidant is decreased inflammation. One study found that diabetics who consumed 125 milliliters of pomegranate juice each day had lower levels of the inflammatory markers C-reactive protein and Interleukin-6 than previously.

Pomegranates are one of the most well-known fruits for increasing libido. Paired with maca root powder, which is known to balance hormones, this Passion Tonic is also an excellent choice for improving your sexual health.

Per Serving
Calories: 154 | Fat: 0.4 g | Protein: 1.4 g | Sodium: 22 mg
Fiber: 1.3 g | Carbohydrates: 36.7 g | Sugar: 32.5 g

GOOD MORNING TONIC

Serves 1

INGREDIENTS

Juice from ½ medium lemon
1 cup warm or room temperature water

1 Pour the lemon juice into the water and stir to combine.
2 Consume immediately, preferably upon waking in the morning.

KEY INGREDIENT: Lemon

You most often hear of the rich amount of vitamin C in lemons, but did you know they are also full of folate, vitamin B_6, magnesium, calcium, phosphorus, and vitamins A and E? Lemon juice is also a natural solvent that attacks the uric acid that causes joint pain and inflammation.

In addition to its anti-inflammatory benefits, there are a number of reasons why drinking lemon water in the morning is a good idea. Drinking lemon water first thing in the morning can help get your body ready for digesting food throughout the day. Lemon water is hydrating and can flush the digestive system, a good idea first thing in the morning. There is evidence that lemon juice can help stimulate proper stomach acid and bile production. This flushing of the digestive system is good for clear skin, and the vitamin C content of lemon juice helps with collagen production.

Per Serving
Calories: 3 | Fat: 0.0 g | Protein: 0.1 g | Sodium: 0 mg
Fiber: 0.1 g | Carbohydrates: 1.1 g | Sugar: 0.4 g

SLEEPING BEAUTY TONIC

Serves 1

INGREDIENTS

1 cup tart cherry juice
1 tablespoon apple cider vinegar
1 tablespoon raw honey

1 Combine cherry juice and apple cider vinegar in a glass.

2 Add the raw honey and stir until dissolved.

3 Consume immediately.

KEY INGREDIENT: Tart Cherries

Tart cherries are working double duty in this tonic. First, they fight inflammation thanks to the anthocyanins they contain. Tart cherries actually have a unique blend of anthocyanins that aren't present in other anthocyanin-rich fruits, even blueberries! Tart cherry juice was specifically studied for its pain-reducing qualities. Runners who drank tart cherry juice reported less pain after races than those who did not drink it, and they also had significantly lower inflammation biomarkers.

In addition to their inflammation-fighting powers, tart cherries are also known to be an incredible sleep aid. Tart cherries are a natural source of melatonin, a hormone responsible for regulating the sleep-wake cycle. This tonic would be an excellent one to include in your daily routine, as regular consumption of tart cherry juice is shown to help people fall asleep faster and sleep longer. In fact, researchers have discovered that drinking tart cherry juice two times daily can increase sleep time by up to ninety minutes!

Per Serving
Calories: 206 | Fat: 0.0 g | Protein: 1.1 g | Sodium: 15 mg
Fiber: 0.0 g | Carbohydrates: 51.4 g | Sugar: 42.3 g

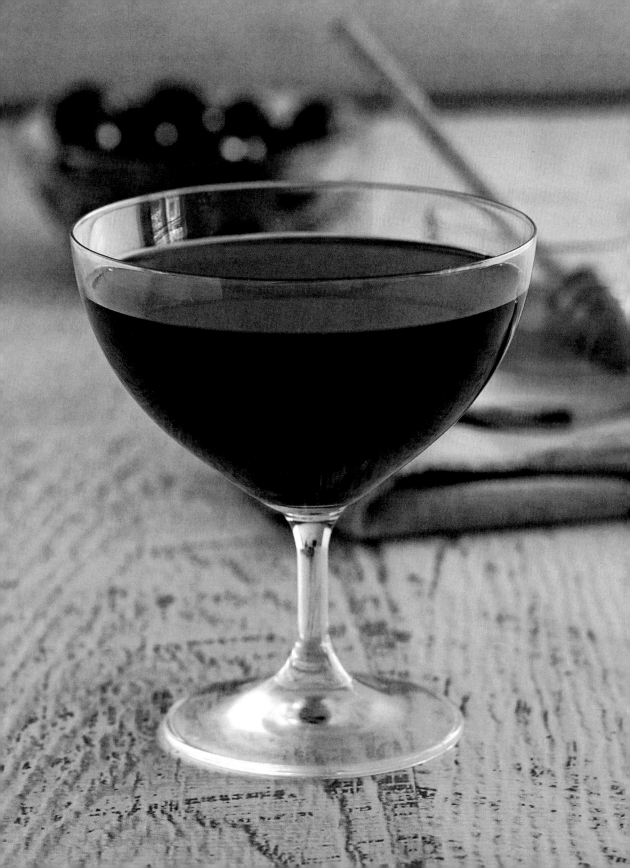

HEALTHY HYDRATION TONIC

Serves 1

INGREDIENTS

½ medium cucumber, cut into chunks
1 large strawberry, hulled and cut in half
½ cup coconut water
Ice, as needed

1 In a small blender, combine the cucumber, strawberry, and coconut water.

2 Blend the ingredients on high until thoroughly combined and smooth.

3 Strain through a fine-mesh sieve. Serve over ice.

4 Consume immediately or store in an airtight container in the refrigerator for 24 hours.

KEY INGREDIENT: Cucumber

Cucumbers are a natural fit for drink recipes. Cucumbers contain up to 95 percent water, so they can help keep you hydrated. Even with all that water, cucumbers contain a good number of nutrients, including vitamin K, B vitamins, copper, potassium, vitamin C, and manganese.

Cucumbers help you fight inflammation in a number of ways. Cucumbers contain an anti-inflammatory flavonoid called *fisetin*. It's been found that fisetin inhibits the pro-inflammatory enzyme cyclooxegynase-2 and inhibits the activation of mitogen-activated protein kinase. In addition, cucumbers contain quercetin. Studies show that quercetin can reduce inflammation by down-regulating nitric oxide synthesis expression.

This tonic recipe contains hydrating, nutritious ingredients and is great to include in your day when you're especially dehydrated or going to be in a situation that warrants extra hydration.

Per Serving
Calories: 45 | Fat: 0.4 g | Protein: 2.0 g | Sodium: 129 mg
Fiber: 0.4 g | Carbohydrates: 9.4 g | Sugar: 6.4 g

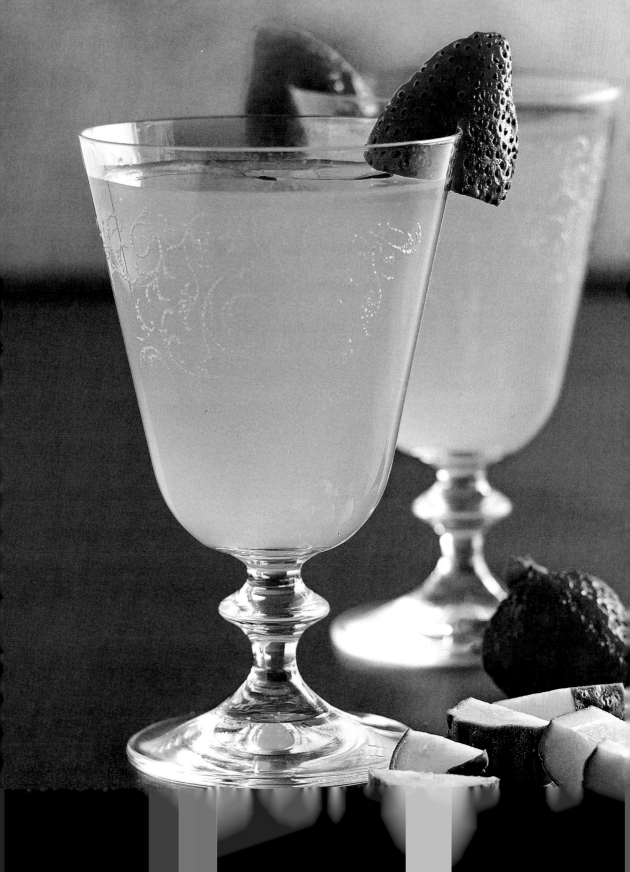

BERRY BEAUTY TONIC

Serves 1

INGREDIENTS

1 cup unsweetened coconut water
½ cup blueberries
1 teaspoon acai berry powder
2 tablespoons lemon juice
¼ teaspoon pure stevia powder
Ice, as needed

1 Place all ingredients except ice in a large blender.
2 Blend the ingredients on high until thoroughly combined and smooth.
3 Fill a large glass with ice and pour the drink over the ice.
4 Consume immediately.

KEY INGREDIENT: Acai Berry Powder

Acai berries have long been a staple in the diet of Indian tribes, but in recent years they have grown in popularity as a superfood health-conscious individuals want to include in their diets also. One reason is that acai is filled with antioxidants such as anthocyanins; polyphenols; and vitamins A, C, and E. It's also a good source of B vitamins, magnesium, potassium, phosphorus, manganese, iron, copper, calcium, and zinc.

The anti-inflammatory properties acai berries boast are due to the combination of antioxidants. Many of the antioxidant compounds found in acai berries have been shown to block inflammatory pathways in the body.

Those same antioxidants make this a potent tonic for beautiful hair and skin. The acai berry's high number of antioxidants makes it helpful for skin regeneration and preventing early signs of aging.

Per Serving
Calories: 111 | Fat: 2.2 g | Protein: 2.4 g | Sodium: 254 mg
Fiber: 6.0 g | Carbohydrates: 23.3 g | Sugar: 14.1 g

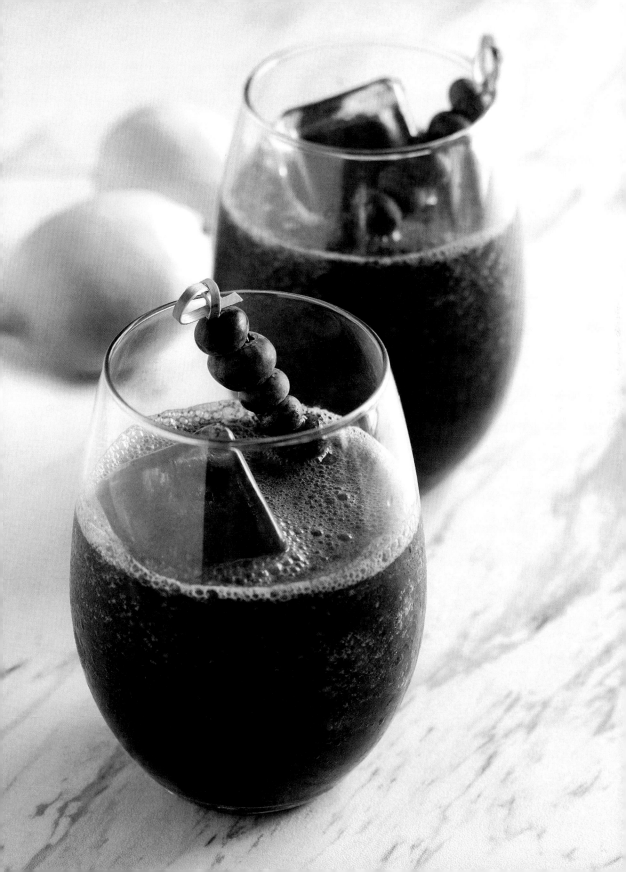

ANTIAGING TONIC

Serves 1

INGREDIENTS

1 cup unsweetened pomegranate juice

1 teaspoon dried amla powder

---

1 Add the pomegranate juice to a small glass.

2 Stir in the amla powder until it is dissolved.

3 Consume immediately.

KEY INGREDIENT: Amla Powder

The list of health benefits associated with amla, also known as *Indian gooseberry*, is long. It's high in vitamin C, phosphorus, calcium, iron, and vitamin B complex. Amla has been associated with aiding hair growth, improving eyesight, lowering the risk of macular degeneration, boosting immunity, treating menstrual cramps, and helping control diabetes. It's also great for controlling chronic and acute inflammation. Studies have shown that consuming amla powder results in similar anti-inflammatory effects as taking anti-inflammatory drugs.

Amla is full of antioxidants that are effective in reducing cellular damage that results from aging. Paired with another potent antioxidant fruit, pomegranate, this makes a powerful antiaging tonic. Look for dried amla powder in your local health food store. It is also readily available online.

Per Serving

Calories: 137 | Fat: 0.4 g | Protein: 0.4 g | Sodium: 22 mg
Fiber: 0.3 g | Carbohydrates: 33.7 g | Sugar: 31.5 g

FIRECRACKER DETOX TONIC

Serves 1

INGREDIENTS

1½ cups water
1 tablespoon apple cider vinegar
1 tablespoon lemon juice
¼ teaspoon ground cinnamon
¼ teaspoon ground ginger
⅛ teaspoon cayenne pepper
1 teaspoon raw honey

1 In a small saucepan, combine the water, apple cider vinegar, lemon juice, cinnamon, ginger, and cayenne pepper over medium heat.

2 Heat the ingredients until they are warm, stirring constantly.

3 Pour into a mug and stir in the raw honey. Serve warm.

4 Consume immediately.

KEY INGREDIENT: Cayenne Pepper

Cayenne pepper is often used to add spiciness to cooking but less often is considered for its health benefits. That should change, though, because cayenne pepper brings a lot of health-promoting properties to the table. It can help digestion and upset stomach; relieve gas, diarrhea, and cramps; improve poor circulation; and even help lower cholesterol. The healing powers of cayenne pepper can be attributed to a compound it contains called *capsaicin*. Capsaicin has anti-inflammatory effects because it inhibits the enzyme activity of COX-2 in the body.

The cayenne pepper gives the heat to this Firecracker Detox Tonic. All of the ingredients work together to aid your body in the natural detox process. This is an exceptional tonic with which to start or end each day.

Per Serving
Calories: 29 | Fat: 0.1 g | Protein: 0.2 g | Sodium: 0 mg
Fiber: 0.5 g | Carbohydrates: 8.0 g | Sugar: 6.3 g

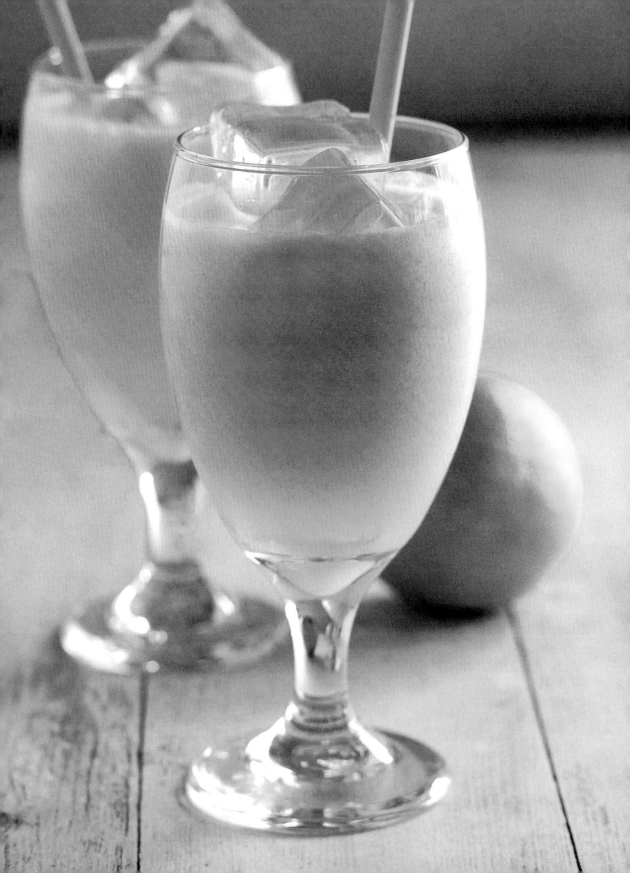

MUSCLE CRAMP RELIEF TONIC

Serves 1

INGREDIENTS

1 cup unsweetened coconut water
¼ cup lite canned coconut milk
1 medium orange, peeled
2 tablespoons baobab fruit powder
Ice, as needed

1 Place all ingredients except
   ice in a large blender.

2 Blend the ingredients on high
   until thoroughly combined and
   smooth.

3 Fill a large glass with ice and
   pour the drink over the ice.

4 Consume immediately or store
   in an airtight container in the
   refrigerator up to 24 hours.

KEY INGREDIENT: Baobab

Baobab is a traditional African medicinal plant. In its native environment it is called "the tree of life." Baobab fruit grows in pods and has a tart, sweet taste. The pulp is taken out and turned into a powder that is worth seeking out. Dried baobab fruit powder is rich in antioxidants, magnesium, potassium, calcium, and protein. The fiber in baobab fruit powder acts as a prebiotic, which helps maintain healthy bacteria in the gut and helps keep inflammation in control.

Mineral depletion can lead to muscle cramping, so eating foods rich in minerals can help prevent muscle cramps. Baobab fruit is high in key minerals thought to play a critical role in relieving muscle cramps: potassium, calcium, and magnesium. Paired with the electrolytes found in coconut water, this tonic is perfect for athletes and highly active individuals.

Per Serving
Calories: 181 | Fat: 4.0 g | Protein: 2.8 g | Sodium: 255 mg
Fiber: 12.2 g | Carbohydrates: 36.2 g | Sugar: 22.8 g

HERBAL DIGESTIVE TONIC

Serves 1

INGREDIENTS

5 mint leaves
2 sage leaves
1 sprig rosemary
1 teaspoon peeled, chopped fresh
   ginger
1 cup plain, unsweetened kombucha

---

1   In a medium bowl, muddle
    together the mint leaves, sage
    leaves, rosemary, and ginger.

2   Add the kombucha to the
    muddled ingredients.

3   Strain through a fine-mesh
    sieve.

4   Consume immediately.

KEY INGREDIENT: Kombucha

When you think of bacteria, you may think of it as a cause of getting sick. It's important to realize, however, that there is good bacteria and bad bacteria. In fact, each of us has a complex ecosystem of bacteria within our bodies known as our *microbiome*. Most of the bacteria lives in our digestive system. Some scientists believe that up to 90 percent of disease can be traced back to the gut and the health of the microbiome. Our food choices play an important role in maintaining the health of our microbiome. Having the right amount of good bacteria and a healthy microbiome has a big part in fighting chronic inflammation. Kombucha is a probiotic-rich beverage that helps promote good bacteria in the gut, thus helping fight inflammation.

Kombucha is also known to help digestion through its unique combination of organic acids, enzymes, and probiotics. The herbs in this drink are also specifically chosen for their digestive properties.

Per Serving
Calories: 31 | Fat: 0.1 g | Protein: 0.1 g | Sodium: 10 mg
Fiber: 0.2 g | Carbohydrates: 7.5 g | Sugar: 2.0 g

COLD-BUSTING SHOT

Serves 1

INGREDIENTS

1 clove garlic
2 tablespoons water
1 tablespoon raw honey

---

1 Finely chop the garlic and allow it to sit 10 minutes.

2 Meanwhile, in a small glass, combine the water and honey.

3 Add the chopped garlic to the water and honey mixture.

4 Consume immediately.

KEY INGREDIENT: Garlic

Garlic has been used medicinally for centuries. It has been used to offer protection against cancer, heart disease, and infections. The health benefits of garlic can be attributed to the organosulfur compounds it possesses. Sulfur compounds play a critical role in your health, helping the cellular detoxification system and the health of your joints and connective tissue, as well as with oxygen-related metabolism. One particular organosulfur compound thought to be associated with garlic's anti-inflammatory action is thiacremonone. Thiacremonone is believed to play in important role in controlling inflammation by suppressing inflammatory activity in the body.

Consuming raw garlic is thought to have a powerful effect on fighting the common cold. Take this Cold-Busting Shot one to two times a day when you're feeling under the weather.

Per Serving
Calories: 67 | Fat: 0.0 g | Protein: 0.3 g | Sodium: 0 mg
Fiber: 0.1 g | Carbohydrates: 18.3 g | Sugar: 17.3 g

ENDURANCE-BUILDER SHOT

Serves 1

INGREDIENTS

2 tablespoons coconut water
1 teaspoon spirulina

1 Place the coconut water and spirulina in a small blender.
2 Blend on high until the ingredients are thoroughly combined.
3 Consume immediately.

KEY INGREDIENT: Spirulina

Spirulina is a freshwater blue-green algae that is noted for its exceptional nutritional profile. It's often touted as the world's most nutrient-dense food. One unique characteristic of spirulina is that it's high in protein, especially for a plant food. Even more unique is that 65 percent of spirulina is a *complete* protein, containing all of the amino acids the body needs. It's also one of the best plant sources of iron; it has, ounce for ounce, twenty-six times the amount of calcium as milk, and it is a great source of B vitamins. Spirulina is also a rich source of omega-3 fatty acids and the fatty acid known as gamma linolenic acid, both of which are known for their anti-inflammatory properties.

Studies have shown that spirulina is effective for increasing endurance and reducing muscle damage from exercise. This is a great shot for athletes and fitness buffs to consume daily.

Per Serving
Calories: 11 | Fat: 0.2 g | Protein: 1.6 g | Sodium: 55 mg
Fiber: 0.4 g | Carbohydrates: 1.7 g | Sugar: 0.8 g

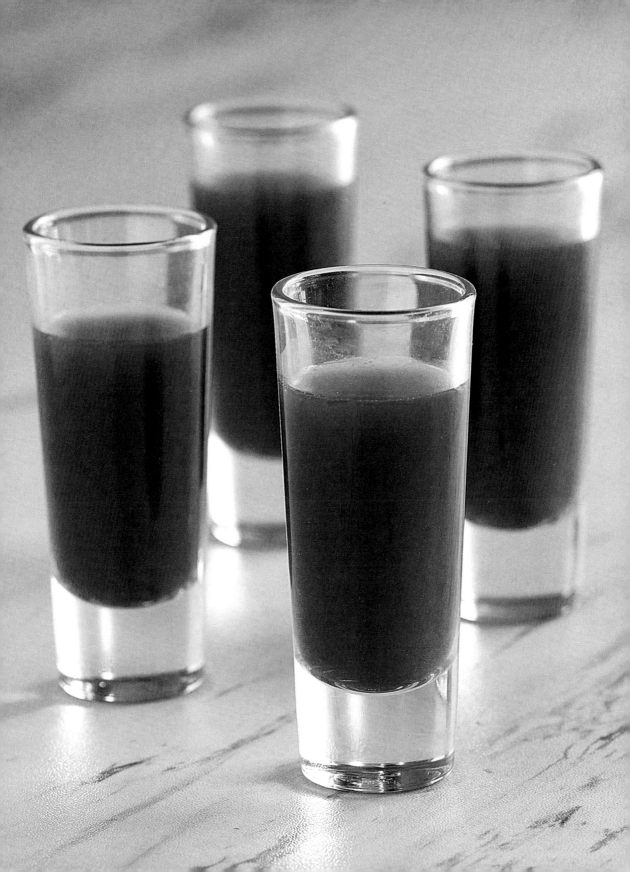

APPLE CIDER VINEGAR SHOT

Serves 1
INGREDIENTS

1 tablespoon apple cider vinegar
2 tablespoons water

1 In a small glass, combine the apple cider vinegar and water.
2 Consume immediately.

KEY INGREDIENT: Apple Cider Vinegar

Apple cider vinegar is made from fermenting apples. This process develops prebiotics, which feed the good bacteria in your gut. This helps maintain a healthy microbiome, which can reduce overall inflammation in the body.

Taking a shot of apple cider vinegar, diluted with water, every day is a healthy habit to maintain. Apple cider vinegar has been shown to have a myriad of health benefits. In addition to its ability to help your body fight inflammation, it can help regulate blood sugar levels, improve skin health, lower cholesterol levels, reduce blood pressure, and relieve symptoms of acid reflux.

Per Serving
Calories: 3 | Fat: 0.0 g | Protein: 0.0 g | Sodium: 0 mg
Fiber: 0.0 g | Carbohydrates: 0.1 g | Sugar: 0.1 g

WHEATGRASS SHOT

Serves 2
INGREDIENTS

1 medium Granny Smith apple
1 cup packed wheatgrass (approximately 25 grams)

1 Prepare the apple by coring it and cutting it into appropriate-sized pieces for your juicer.
2 Process the apple and wheatgrass through the juicer.
3 Consume immediately or store in a glass airtight container in the refrigerator up to 12 hours if using a centrifugal juicer and up to 3 days if using a masticating juicer.

KEY INGREDIENT: Wheatgrass

Wheatgrass is a type of young grass in the wheat family. Despite the name, wheatgrass is a gluten-free edible grass. It's often consumed for its health benefits because it's a concentrated source of a number of important nutrients. You will find iron; calcium; magnesium; amino acids; and vitamins A, C, and E in wheatgrass. Wheatgrass is also one of the world's richest forms of chlorophyll. Chlorophyll has been shown to be effective against cancer, to help protect against the hazards of radiation, to be antimicrobial, and to be effective for wound healing. Studies have shown that wheatgrass has significant anti-inflammatory activity in cases of chronic inflammation. This Wheatgrass Shot is a good daily, overall health-promoting shot.

Per Serving
Calories: 43 | Fat: 0.0 g | Protein: 0.4 g | Sodium: 1 mg
Fiber: 0.0 g | Carbohydrates: 9.2 g | Sugar: 8.0 g

HANGOVER CURE SHOT

Serves 1

INGREDIENTS

1 medium beet
1 teaspoon peeled, coarsely
  chopped fresh ginger

1 Prepare the beet by peeling it
   and cutting it into appropriate-
   sized pieces for your juicer.

2 Process the beet and ginger
   through the juicer. Do not
   strain.

3 Consume immediately. Can
   be stored in an airtight container in the refrigerator up to
   12 hours if using a centrifugal
   juicer and up to 3 days if using
   a masticating juicer.

KEY INGREDIENT: Beets

While beets are an anti-inflammatory food, there are other health benefits that come along with eating (or juicing) beets. The same unique phytonutrient that helps beets be a potent anti-inflammatory agent, betaine, makes this vegetable a great choice if you've drunk too much alcohol. The betaine pigments are what give beets their bright crimson color, and they also help facilitate the body's natural detoxification process. They trigger the detoxification process and aid in the elimination of toxins.

While the beet helps eliminate toxins in this recipe, the ginger will help with upset stomach. If you're feeling the effects of alcohol, this is a good shot to turn to.

Per Serving
Calories: 31 | Fat: 0.0 g | Protein: 1.4 g | Sodium: 63 mg
Fiber: 0.0 g | Carbohydrates: 5.9 g | Sugar: 5.6 g

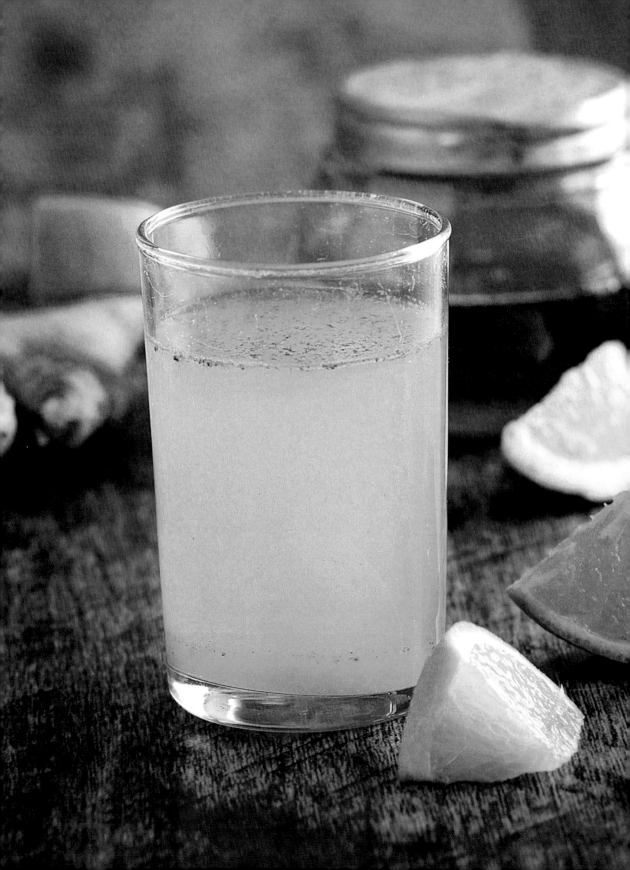

IMMUNITY-BOOSTER SHOT

Serves 1

INGREDIENTS

1 small orange, peeled
½ teaspoon peeled, chopped fresh ginger
½ teaspoon raw honey
⅛ teaspoon cayenne powder

---

1 Using a citrus press or your hands, squeeze the juice from the orange into the container of a small blender. It should yield approximately ¼ cup juice.

2 Add ginger, raw honey, and cayenne powder to the blender and blend on high until all ingredients are thoroughly combined and smooth.

3 Consume immediately.

KEY INGREDIENT: Raw Honey

The medicinal value of honey has been known since ancient times. It was often used as an ointment and wound healing agent because of its antimicrobial properties. Aristotle noted that honey was "good as a salve for sore eyes and wounds." In modern times, honey's ability to assist with wound healing has been demonstrated.

Even though honey consists of mainly sugar and water, it also contains vitamins, minerals, and antioxidants. The antioxidants help prevent oxidative damages that can lead to inflammation. Recent studies have also shown that honey inhibits the activity of pro-inflammatory COX-2.

Honey that's been heated can lose a lot of its health benefits, so it's important to use raw, unprocessed honey.

The immunity-boosting ingredients in this shot make it useful at the very first signs of sickness.

Per Serving
Calories: 37 | Fat: 0.1 g | Protein: 0.5 g | Sodium: 0 mg
Fiber: 0.2 g | Carbohydrates: 9.7 g | Sugar: 8.2 g

ELDERBERRY SYRUP SHOT

Serves 32

INGREDIENTS

¾ cup dried elderberries

3 cups water

1 cinnamon stick

4 whole cloves

1 tablespoon peeled, chopped fresh ginger

1 cup raw honey

---

1 In a large pot, bring the elderberries, water, cinnamon stick, cloves, and ginger to a boil.

2 Reduce the heat to medium-low, cover, and simmer until the liquid has reduced by half, about 30–40 minutes.

3 Allow the liquid to cool, then strain through a fine-mesh sieve.

4 Press all the liquid out of the berries using the back of a wooden spoon.

5 Add the raw honey and stir until combined.

6 Store in an airtight container in the refrigerator up to 2 months. Recommended 1 tablespoon shot daily as a preventative measure and up to 2–3 shots daily when ill.

KEY INGREDIENT: Elderberries

Elderberries are grown in the United States and were traditionally used by Native Americans, who benefited from every part of the plant. Elderberries are found in a number of Native American folk remedies and are used for relieving cold and flu symptoms, reducing congestion, alleviating arthritis pain, treating upset stomach and gas, and promoting healthy detoxification. Research has shown that, indeed, consuming the extract of elderberries helps reduce the duration of the flu by three days! Elderberries are a good source of vitamins A, C, and B_6; potassium; and iron. In addition, elderberries are antioxidant rich, which could contribute to their anti-inflammatory properties.

Elderberry syrup is used both as a preventative measure to prevent illness and also to shorten its duration. It's best taken every day during the cold and flu season.

Per Serving

Calories: 34 | Fat: 0.0 g | Protein: 0.1 g | Sodium: 0 mg
Fiber: 0.0 g | Carbohydrates: 9.3 g | Sugar: 8.7 g

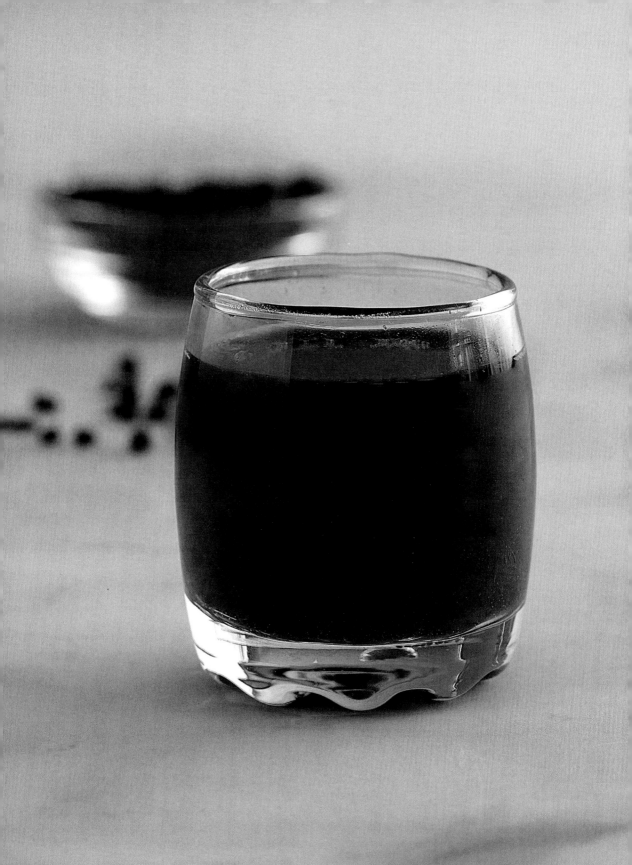

PREGAME SHOT

Serves 2

INGREDIENTS

3 baby radicchio leaves
1 medium pink or red grapefruit

---

1 Prepare the radicchio leaves by chopping them into appropriate-sized pieces for your juicer.

2 Prepare the grapefruit by removing the peel and cutting the fruit into appropriate-sized pieces for your juicer.

3 Process the radicchio leaves and grapefruit through the juicer.

4 Strain through a fine-mesh sieve if desired.

5 Consume immediately or store in a glass airtight container in the refrigerator up to 12 hours if using a centrifugal juicer and up to 3 days if using a masticating juicer.

KEY INGREDIENT: Radicchio

Radicchio is bitter and, like many bitter foods, it is good for your gut health. In addition to its anti-inflammatory properties, radicchio is an excellent digestive aid. The inulin in radicchio promotes healthy digestion and also helps balance blood sugar levels. Compounds in radicchio stimulate the liver to produce bile, a fluid that helps the body digest fatty foods. This is called Pregame Shot because it's especially helpful to take before consuming a heavy meal.

Per Serving
Calories: 50 | Fat: 0.1 g | Protein: 1.1 g | Sodium: 2 mg
Fiber: 0.0 g | Carbohydrates: 11.6 g | Sugar: 8.6 g

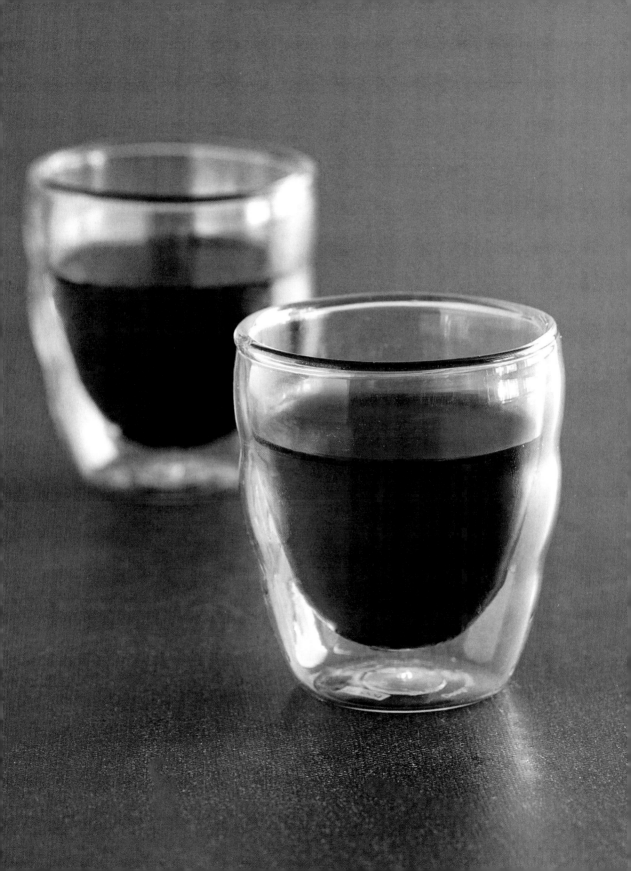

CONGESTION-FIGHTING SHOT

Serves 2

INGREDIENTS

1 small handful young mustard greens
1 teaspoon peeled, coarsely
  chopped ginger

1 Prepare the mustard greens by
   cutting off the ends and chopping them into appropriate-
   sized pieces for your juicer. You
   should have approximately
   2 cups chopped mustard
   greens.

2 Process the mustard greens
   and ginger through the juicer.

3 Strain through a fine-mesh
   sieve if desired.

4 Consume immediately or store
   in a glass airtight container in
   the refrigerator up to 12 hours
   if using a centrifugal juicer and
   up to 3 days if using a masticating juicer.

KEY INGREDIENT: Mustard Greens

Mustard greens are a nutritionally dense vegetable that is especially high in antioxidants, namely vitamin A and vitamin C. Antioxidants help prevent cell damage caused by oxidative stress. When free radicals damage cells, chronic inflammation can result. Therefore, eating foods high in antioxidants is a good way to prevent inflammation in the body. Mustard greens are also extremely high in vitamin K, another critical nutrient for reducing inflammation.

Mustard greens have a spicy mustard flavor and are helpful, along with raw ginger, in helping to relieve congestion. If you often wake up congested, this shot will help clear your airways.

Per Serving
Calories: 6 | Fat: 0.0 g | Protein: 0.8 g | Sodium: 5 mg
Fiber: 0.0 g | Carbohydrates: 0.6 g | Sugar: 0.4 g

IMMUNITY-BOOSTING TONIC

Serves 1

INGREDIENTS

2 medium oranges
1 teaspoon camu camu powder
Ice, as needed

1 Use a citrus juicer or your hands to squeeze the juice from the oranges into a glass.

2 Stir in the camu camu powder until it is completely dissolved.

3 Add ice and consume immediately.

KEY INGREDIENT: Camu Camu Powder

Camu camu is a shrub found in the swamp or flooded areas of the Amazon rainforest. Its berries look similar to cherries and are one of the highest vitamin C foods on the planet. The camu camu berry has ten to sixty times the vitamin C content of an orange! In addition to its extraordinarily high vitamin C content, camu camu also contains manganese, iron, copper, magnesium, calcium, potassium, and zinc. It also contains the carotenoid lutein, known for its anti-inflammatory action. Lutein is shown to inhibit pro-inflammatory proteins in the body.

Camu camu's high vitamin C content makes it a good choice for boosting your immune system function. It has a naturally sour flavor, so it works well with sweeter orange juice. You can find camu camu powder in a health food store or online.

Per Serving
Calories: 94 | Fat: 0.2 g | Protein: 1.2 g | Sodium: 1 mg
Fiber: 0.3 g | Carbohydrates: 21.2 g | Sugar: 13.9 g

GLOWING SKIN SHOT

Serves 1

INGREDIENTS

¼ cup packed cilantro leaves
¼ cup unsweetened coconut water
1 tablespoon lemon juice

---

1 Place all ingredients in a small blender.
2 Blend the ingredients on high until the cilantro is thoroughly broken down and combined with the liquid.
3 Consume immediately.

KEY INGREDIENT: Cilantro

Cilantro has an impressive list of nutrients and health benefits. It's a great source of vitamins A, C, and K and B vitamins. In addition, cilantro provides minerals like potassium, calcium, manganese, iron, and magnesium. It's also high in antioxidants, including superstars like quercetin, kaempferol, rhamnetin, and apigenin. A lot of powerful nutrition is packed into those green leaves!

Research shows that cilantro can help lower cholesterol, lower blood pressure, and support healthy cardiovascular function. It has also been shown to help accelerate the removal of toxins from the body and to prevent neurological inflammation.

Cilantro has natural antihistamines, so this shot is perfect for relief from skin irritations.

Per Serving
Calories: 14 | Fat: 0.2 g | Protein: 0.6 g | Sodium: 64 mg
Fiber: 0.8 g | Carbohydrates: 3.5 g | Sugar: 1.9 g

Chapter 6
HOT DRINKS

From teas to lattes to hot cocoa, hot drinks can warm your body and soul. Sipping on a hot beverage in the afternoon is a ritual I've come to love. It's so common to purchase hot drinks from coffee shops that may taste delicious but don't do you any favors when it comes to your health. Instead of choosing a warm drink that is full of sugar and causes inflammation, why not use foods that fight inflammation and make your own warm, comforting drinks at home? That's exactly what you'll find here.

This chapter covers all of your favorite hot drinks that are made especially with ingredients that will help reduce inflammation. Most of them take just minutes to make and are full of nutritional benefits. It's time to ditch the coffee-shop drinks and make your own anti-inflammatory hot drinks!

MEXICAN HOT CHOCOLATE

Serves 2
INGREDIENTS

1 cup lite canned coconut milk
1½ cups unsweetened almond milk
1 teaspoon ground cinnamon
¼ teaspoon chili powder
1 teaspoon pure vanilla extract
¼ cup pure maple syrup
¼ cup raw cacao powder

1   In a small saucepan over medium-high heat, whisk to combine the coconut milk, almond milk, cinnamon, chili powder, vanilla extract, and maple syrup.

2   Bring the mixture to a boil, reduce the heat, and simmer 5 minutes until it thickens slightly.

3   Whisk in the cacao powder and remove from heat.

4   Serve warm. Store any leftovers in an airtight container in the refrigerator up to 48 hours. May be reheated.

KEY INGREDIENT: Raw Cacao Powder

Cacao beans are high in polyphenols, which work with your body to reduce inflammation. They are shown to have a range of cardiovascular-protective properties and boast *forty times* the antioxidants of blueberries. Another benefit? Cacao is the highest plant-based source of iron. Yes, you're doing your body a big favor by drinking this Mexican Hot Chocolate!

This hot chocolate drink is sweetened with an unrefined, natural sweetener: maple syrup. Maple syrup contains antioxidants and is a rich source of minerals like manganese and zinc. One study showed that maple syrup has twenty-four different antioxidants. These antioxidants can help reduce free radical damage, which causes inflammation.

Per Serving
Calories: 249 | Fat: 10.1 g | Protein: 2.9 g | Sodium: 156 mg
Fiber: 3.6 g | Carbohydrates: 36.9 g | Sugar: 24.4 g

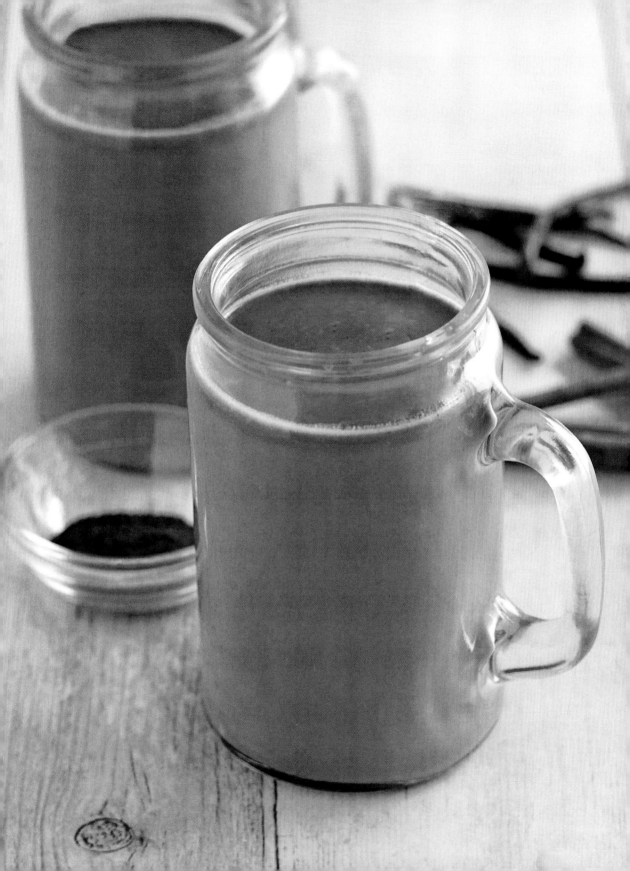

GREEN TEA WITH GINGER AND LEMON

Serves 1

INGREDIENTS

1 cup water
1 tablespoon peeled, chopped fresh
   ginger
1 tablespoon lemon juice
1 teaspoon raw honey
1 tea bag green tea leaves

---

1 In a small saucepan, combine
   the water, ginger, and lemon
   juice and bring to a boil over
   high heat.

2 Remove from heat and strain
   the ginger from the water and
   transfer the water to a teacup.

3 Stir honey into the water until it
   is dissolved.

4 Steep the tea bag in the water
   3 minutes.

5 Consume immediately.

KEY INGREDIENT: Green Tea

Green tea contains quercetin, a chemical compound that has strong anti-inflammatory properties. Green tea is one of the most health-promoting things you can drink. Studies have shown that regularly drinking green tea can help prevent diseases like heart disease and stroke, and consuming it daily is correlated with longer life spans.

Here green tea is paired with fresh ginger for extra protection against inflammation. Lemon juice also provides health benefits along with antioxidant-rich raw honey. Be sure to wait until you remove the water from the heat to add the raw honey so you protect the important enzymes present in the honey.

Per Serving
Calories: 30 | Fat: 0.1 g | Protein: 0.2 g | Sodium: 0 mg
Fiber: 0.2 g | Carbohydrates: 8.7 g | Sugar: 6.3 g

MORNING DETOX TEA

Serves 1

INGREDIENTS

1½ cups water
2 tablespoons lemon juice
1 tablespoon apple cider vinegar
1" piece fresh ginger, peeled and
  sliced
1 teaspoon raw honey

1 In a small saucepan over
   medium heat, combine the
   water, lemon juice, apple cider
   vinegar, and sliced ginger and
   bring to a simmer. Simmer 2
   minutes.

2 Strain the ginger from the
   mixture and pour tea into a
   teacup.

3 Stir in the raw honey.

4 Serve warm immediately or
   store in an airtight container in
   the refrigerator up to 48 hours.
   May be reheated.

KEY INGREDIENT: Fresh Ginger

Ginger is used in a number of recipes in this book, and that's because it's one of the top inflammation-fighting foods. It's evident that it will help your body fight inflammation and is advantageous to include in your diet as often as possible. Ginger has such strong anti-inflammatory properties that it's often used to reduce pain in arthritis patients.

Although our bodies do a great job of naturally detoxing, this morning tea can help that natural process. It contains ingredients that can aid detox, such as lemon juice and apple cider vinegar. This is a lovely and health-promoting way to start each morning!

Per Serving
Calories: 31 | Fat: 0.0 g | Protein: 0.2 g | Sodium: 0 mg
Fiber: 0.2 g | Carbohydrates: 8.5 g | Sugar: 6.7 g

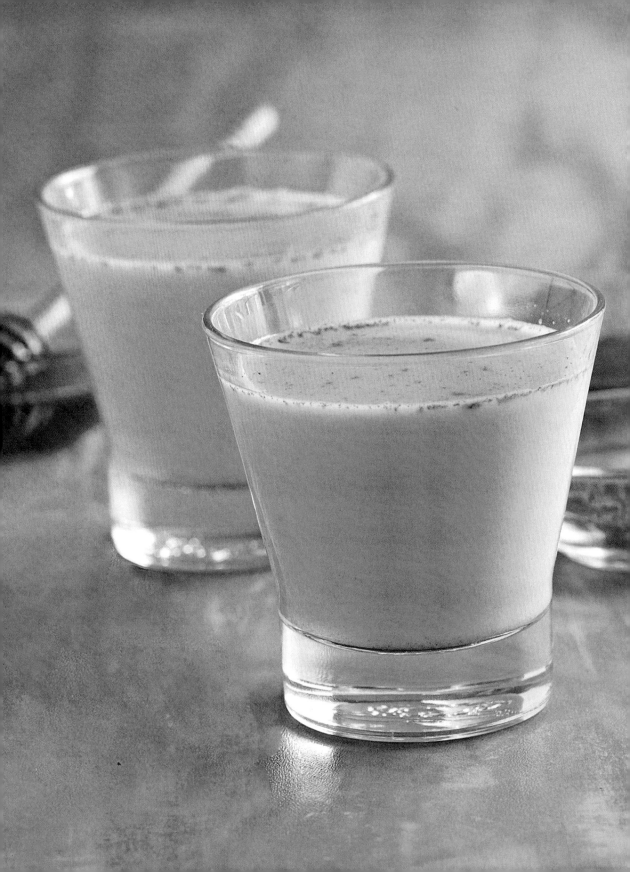

GOLDEN MILK

Serves 2

INGREDIENTS

For the Turmeric Paste

¼ cup turmeric powder
½ cup water
¾ teaspoon black pepper

For the Golden Milk

2 cups unsweetened almond milk
½ teaspoon Turmeric Paste
¼ teaspoon ground cinnamon
¼ teaspoon ground ginger
½ teaspoon pure vanilla extract
½ teaspoon coconut oil
2 teaspoons raw honey

1   First, prepare the Turmeric Paste: Mix the turmeric powder and water in a small saucepan over low heat, stirring until a paste is formed.

2   Once you have a paste, stir in the black pepper.

3   This recipe provides more Turmeric Paste than you'll need for this Golden Milk recipe, so cool and store the extra in a glass jar in the refrigerator up to 2 weeks.

4   Next, combine the almond milk, Turmeric Paste, cinnamon, ginger, vanilla extract, coconut oil, and honey in a small saucepan and gently heat over low heat.

5   Whisk well to ensure you combine the paste, oil, and spices.

6   Serve warm. Store any leftovers in an airtight container in the refrigerator up to 48 hours. May be reheated.

KEY INGREDIENT: Turmeric

Turmeric has been used holistically for centuries. A spice common in India, its bright yellow color gives this hot drink its name. In Southeast Asia, it is so highly regarded that it's used not only as a principle spice but also as a component in religious ceremonies.

Curcumin is the active ingredient that gives turmeric its anti-inflammatory effect. Curcumin isn't easily absorbed by your body; it does better when paired with black pepper, and that's why you find black pepper on the ingredient list for this Turmeric Paste. Some studies also suggest that it's more easily absorbed when consumed with fat, so coconut oil provides that.

Turmeric has gained the attention of many in the modern medicine field, indicated by the fact that it's been the subject of over 3,000 scientific publications in the last twenty-five years. The results of numerous studies prove that turmeric is a powerful anti-inflammatory agent that can be used to help combat a number of inflammatory-related diseases and conditions.

Per Serving

Calories: 65 | Fat: 4.1 g | Protein: 1.1 g | Sodium: 180 mg
Fiber: 1.3 g | Carbohydrates: 8.7 g | Sugar: 6.4 g

PUMPKIN SPICE LATTE

Serves 2

INGREDIENTS

2 cups vanilla walnut milk
½ cup brewed coffee
¼ cup pumpkin purée
2 tablespoons erythritol
1 tablespoon pure vanilla extract
½ teaspoon pumpkin spice

1 Combine all ingredients in a small saucepan.

2 Whisk until all the ingredients are thoroughly combined.

3 Gently heat over medium-low heat, whisking occasionally, until the drink is hot, about 5 minutes.

4 Serve hot. Store in an airtight container in the refrigerator up to 2 days. May be reheated.

KEY INGREDIENT: Pumpkin

Pumpkin-spiced drinks have risen to extreme popularity so much in recent years that if you see the acronym PSL in October, you know exactly what it means. The problem is that most of these Pumpkin Spice Lattes are made without any real pumpkin at all and are filled with inflammatory ingredients like dairy and refined sugar. You can make a much healthier, anti-inflammatory Pumpkin Spice Latte at home with this simple recipe.

By adding pumpkin purée (canned works just fine) to your latte, you're adding a good amount of fiber, vitamin A, vitamin C, vitamin B_6, copper, and manganese. Pumpkin boasts a high level of the antioxidant beta-carotene. Beta-carotene is known to help protect eye health, improve respiratory health, and protect the body from free radical damage. That protection also helps keep inflammation at bay.

Per Serving
Calories: 92 | Fat: 3.7 g | Protein: 1.4 g | Sodium: 142 mg
Fiber: 1.8 g | Carbohydrates: 20.6 g | Sugar: 6.1 g
Sugar Alcohol: 12.0 g

COFFEE, ELEVATED

Serves 1

INGREDIENTS

1 cup brewed coffee
1 tablespoon coconut oil

---

1 Pour hot, brewed coffee into a mug.

2 Add the coconut oil and stir until it is melted into the coffee.

3 Consume immediately.

KEY INGREDIENT: Coconut Oil

Coconut oil can be confusing, as there is a lot of contradictory information you can find as to whether it's beneficial for your health or not. While coconut oil is composed of saturated fats, it has a special kind of fats called *medium chain fatty acids*. These unique fats include caprylic acid, lauric acid, and capric acid. One indication that these medium chain fatty acids are beneficial is that lauric acid is one of the primary lipids found in breast milk. Medium chain fatty acids have been shown to be beneficial for brain, skin, immune system, and thyroid health.

Coconut oil is at work here to fight inflammation. The lauric acid in coconut oil has anti-inflammatory properties. Some studies have shown it to reduce inflammation better than leading medications.

Per Serving
Calories: 119 | Fat: 12.8 g | Protein: 0.3 g | Sodium: 4 mg
Fiber: 0.0 g | Carbohydrates: 0.0 g | Sugar: 0.0 g

MATCHA VANILLA LATTE

Serves 1
INGREDIENTS

¼ cup hot water
1 teaspoon matcha powder
1 cup lite canned coconut milk
¼ teaspoon pure stevia powder
⅛ teaspoon ground cinnamon
¼ teaspoon pure vanilla extract
2 teaspoons raw honey

1 Mix together the hot water and matcha powder in a coffee mug until the matcha is dissolved.

2 In a small saucepan over medium-low heat, whisk together the coconut milk, stevia powder, cinnamon, and vanilla extract. Heat until the mixture is hot, 2–3 minutes.

3 Pour the coconut milk mixture into the coffee mug with the matcha. Stir in the raw honey until dissolved.

4 Consume immediately.

KEY INGREDIENT: Matcha

Matcha, consumed in Japan for almost 1,000 years, was traditionally reserved for royalty and spiritual leaders. Today it is widely available at most supermarkets and is the only tea where you consume the whole tea leaf. This unique fact is what makes it special and abundant in health benefits.

Matcha is an antioxidant powerhouse, surpassing even the most antioxidant-rich foods like blueberries and dark chocolate. Although the mechanisms are not yet fully understood, the antioxidants in matcha, called *catechins*, are shown to have strong anti-inflammatory effects. Matcha is also known as an anti-inflammatory agent partly because of the chlorophyll it contains. Matcha is five times higher than regular green tea in chlorophyll, which interferes with the growth of bacterial-induced inflammation.

Matcha is also fantastic for sustained energy throughout the day thanks to L-theanine, an amino acid found in all green teas. It has also been found to have a calming effect for people who suffer from anxiety, as it binds to the same brain cell receptors as glutamate, producing an inhibitory effect.

Although matcha has an earthy flavor, it is masked with vanilla, coconut milk, cinnamon, honey, and stevia in this tasty latte.

Per Serving
Calories: 200 | Fat: 13.5 g | Protein: 0.6 g | Sodium: 15 mg
Fiber: 0.7 g | Carbohydrates: 16.0 g | Sugar: 11.7 g

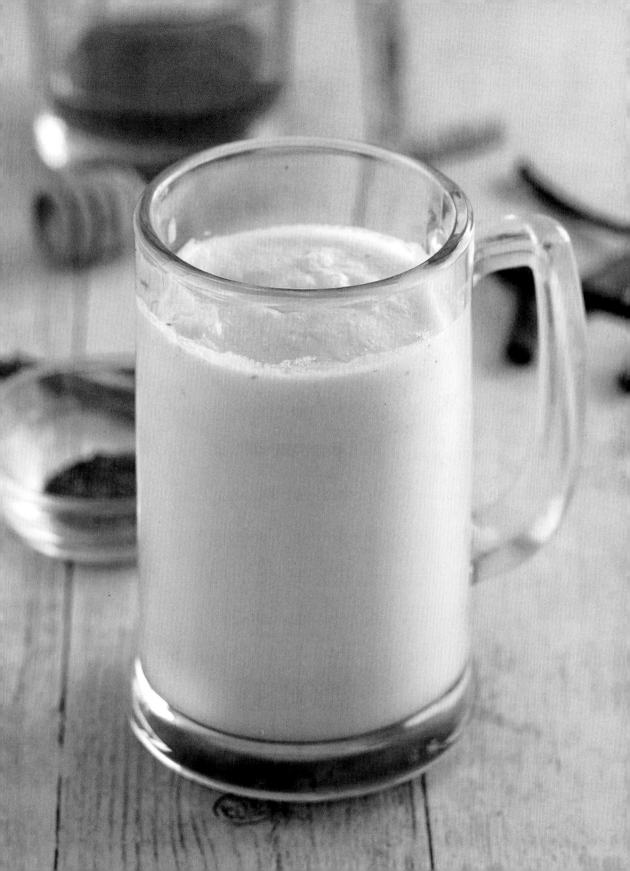

CLOVE TEA

Serves 1

INGREDIENTS

1 tablespoon whole dried cloves
1 cup water
1 teaspoon pure maple syrup

---

1 Using a mortar and pestle, coarsely grind the whole cloves.

2 Combine the coarsely ground cloves and water in a small saucepan over medium-high heat and bring to a boil. Turn off heat immediately after the mixture boils.

3 Cover the pan. Allow to steep 3 minutes.

4 Strain through a fine-mesh strainer into a mug.

5 Stir in maple syrup.

6 Consume immediately.

KEY INGREDIENT: Cloves

Cloves are the dried flower buds of the Syzygium aromaticum tree. In the culinary world, they are a wonderful spice that brings a unique, warming flavor to whatever they are added to. Not only do they have fantastic sweet and spicy flavor, but they also have tremendous health benefits. Cloves have been shown to have antifungal, antiviral, antioxidant, anticancer, and anti-inflammatory properties. Eugenol is the compound at work fighting inflammation. It works, similar to many anti-inflammatory compounds, by blocking pro-inflammatory COX-2.

This Clove Tea, which pairs perfectly with maple syrup, is a lovely way to enjoy all the health benefits of cloves.

Per Serving
Calories: 32 | Fat: 0.6 g | Protein: 0.4 g | Sodium: 18 mg
Fiber: 1.2 g | Carbohydrates: 7.7 g | Sugar: 4.1 g

GINGERBREAD LATTE

Serves 1

INGREDIENTS

¼ cup full-fat coconut milk
1 teaspoon blackstrap molasses
¼ teaspoon pure stevia powder
Pinch ground cinnamon
Pinch ground ginger
Pinch allspice
Pinch ground nutmeg
1 cup brewed hot coffee

1 In a small saucepan, whisk together the coconut milk, blackstrap molasses, stevia, cinnamon, ginger, allspice, and nutmeg.

2 Heat the milk mixture over medium-low heat until it is warm, about 5 minutes, whisking frequently.

3 Pour the coffee into a mug and stir in the milk mixture.

4 Consume immediately.

KEY INGREDIENT: Coffee

Those of you who love your morning cup of coffee will be pleased to hear that it's more than just a way to help you wake up. Coffee brings a number of health benefits. Studies have shown that drinking coffee is associated with a lower risk for Alzheimer's disease and Parkinson's disease, and it even lowers the risk of some types of cancer. In two large studies over an eighteen- to twenty-four–year period, coffee was also associated with living longer, showing a 20 percent lower risk of death among men who drank coffee and a 26 percent lower risk of death among women who drank coffee.

Coffee is a rich source of polyphenols, powerful antioxidants. It is the polyphenols that are believed to bring coffee its anti-inflammatory benefits.

Per Serving
Calories: 133 | Fat: 11.4 g | Protein: 1.5 g | Sodium: 13 mg
Fiber: 0.2 g | Carbohydrates: 7.2 g | Sugar: 5.3 g

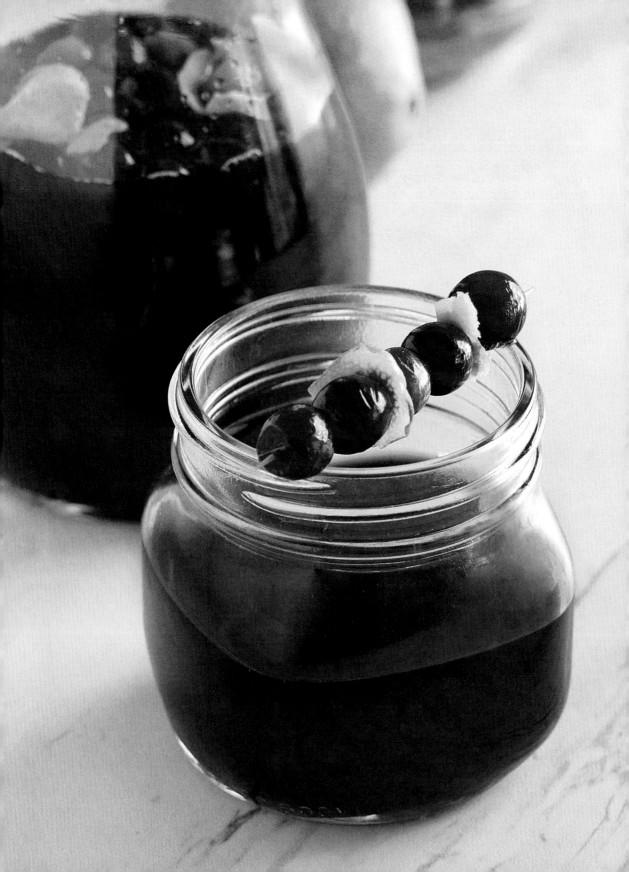

SPICED CRANBERRY DRINK

Serves 4

INGREDIENTS

3 cups whole cranberries
1 cup fresh orange juice
4 cups water
1 cinnamon stick
2 whole cloves
⅓ cup pure maple syrup
⅓ cup erythritol

---

1 Combine all ingredients in a large pot and bring to a boil.

2 Reduce the heat and allow the ingredients to simmer, stirring occasionally, for 20 minutes.

3 Strain the ingredients through a fine-mesh strainer, using the back of a wooden spoon to push the juice from the remaining cranberries.

4 Serve warm. Store in an airtight container in the refrigerator up to 4 days. May be reheated.

KEY INGREDIENT: Cranberries

Cranberries are rich in antioxidants known to fight inflammation. In addition to powerful anthocyanins, cranberries are also a good source of vitamin C and vitamin E. Studies have shown that consuming cranberries increases the total antioxidant capacity in the bloodstream.

Inflammation and oxidative stress in the body both have detrimental effects on your cardiovascular health. The ability of cranberries to fight inflammation and oxidation through the presence of antioxidants makes them excellent at protecting cardiovascular health.

This Spiced Cranberry Drink is an excellent fall and winter drink that would be a wonderful addition to holiday gatherings. It is sweetened naturally with erythritol, and fresh orange juice and pure maple syrup also add a natural sweetness. The orange juice provides extra vitamin C as well, making this an exceptionally nutritious drink recipe.

Per Serving
Calories: 123 | Fat: 0.1 g | Protein: 0.7 g | Sodium: 5 mg
Fiber: 0.6 g | Carbohydrates: 45.6 g | Sugar: 24.1 g
Sugar Alcohol: 16.0 g

COLLAGEN COFFEE

Serves 1

INGREDIENTS

1 cup hot brewed coffee
2 tablespoons plain collagen protein
  powder

1 Pour the coffee into a mug.
2 Stir in the collagen protein until
  it is dissolved.
3 Consume immediately.

KEY INGREDIENT: Collagen Protein

Collagen is the most abundant protein in your body. As you age, your body's natural collagen production slows down. Today, animal collagen is available in powdered form, allowing you to replace lost collagen in your body and reap the health benefits. Consuming collagen (not using it topically in beauty products but actually ingesting it) is associated with improving the health of the skin, hair, nails, and teeth; reducing joint pain and degeneration; and protecting your cardiovascular health. Studies have demonstrated the anti-inflammatory properties of collagen. One study reported that collagen was 25 percent more effective than standard anti-inflammatory drugs at reducing joint pain.

Plain collagen powder is odorless and tasteless, so adding collagen to your morning coffee is an easy way to add it to your daily routine.

Per Serving
Calories: 38 | Fat: 0.0 g | Protein: 9.3 g | Sodium: 58 mg
Fiber: 0.0 g | Carbohydrates: 0.0 g | Sugar: 0.0 g

REISHI MUSHROOM COFFEE

Serves 4

INGREDIENTS

For the Reishi Mushroom Tea
8 cups water
1 cup dried reishi mushroom pieces

For the Reishi Mushroom Coffee
4 cups hot brewed coffee

---

1 Start by making Reishi Mushroom Tea: Bring water to a boil in a medium saucepan.

2 Add the reishi mushroom pieces to the water and boil 30 minutes.

3 Turn off the heat, cover the pan, and allow to steep 15 minutes.

4 Remove the dried mushroom pieces and transfer the Reishi Mushroom Tea to an airtight container. The tea can be kept in the refrigerator up to 1 week.

5 To make each serving of the Reishi Mushroom Coffee, add ½ cup warm Reishi Mushroom Tea to 1 cup of hot brewed coffee.

6 Consume immediately.

KEY INGREDIENT: Reishi Mushrooms

Native to Asia, the reishi mushroom is an edible, medicinal fungus that's been used for thousands of years for its healing properties. Reishi mushroom is considered an adaptogen herb, which means it can help your body deal with the negative effects of stress. One such effect of stress is inflammation; therefore, reishi mushrooms are a powerful way to fight inflammation.

In addition to fighting inflammation, the reishi mushroom has been noted for its ability to fight fatigue, skin disorders, viruses, tumors, autoimmune disorders, heart disease, and sleeping disorders. Talk about a potent ingredient to include in your diet!

Alone, reishi mushroom tea is quite bitter and doesn't have a pleasant taste. Mixing it with coffee solves the problem and makes it easier to drink. Feel free to drink it alone, however, if you like the flavor!

Per Serving
Calories: 4 | Fat: 0.0 g | Protein: 0.4 g | Sodium: 4 mg
Fiber: 0.0 g | Carbohydrates: 0.5 g | Sugar: 0.0 g

TART CHERRY TURMERIC BEDTIME TEA

Serves 1

INGREDIENTS

1 cup tart cherry juice
1 cup water
1 tablespoon grated fresh turmeric
Pinch black pepper
Pinch ground cinnamon
1 chamomile tea bag
1 teaspoon raw honey

1 In a small saucepan, combine the tart cherry juice, water, turmeric, black pepper, and cinnamon.

2 Bring to a simmer over medium heat. Allow to simmer 5–7 minutes, until the liquid reduces by almost half.

3 Strain the mixture through a fine-mesh strainer and pour into a mug with the chamomile tea bag.

4 Allow the tea to brew 3 minutes.

5 Remove the tea bag and stir in the raw honey.

6 Consume immediately.

KEY INGREDIENT: Tart Cherry

Cherries have one of the highest levels of anti-inflammatory fighting power among foods. Specifically, the anthocyanins in cherries (the antioxidant compound in cherries that also gives them their bright red color) have been linked to reduce inflammation at levels compared to some pain medications. Cherries have also shown promise in treating arthritis and osteoarthritis—both conditions caused by inflammation—and in reducing the amount of circulating concentrations of inflammatory biomarkers in the blood.

Since the early twenty-first century the tart cherry has been promoted for its health benefits. Because of its positive effects on sleep quality and duration, this tea is perfect to drink before bedtime. In addition to helping you sleep, this Tart Cherry Turmeric Bedtime Tea is filled with inflammation-fighting ingredients.

Per Serving
Calories: 190 | Fat: 0.3 g | Protein: 2.0 g | Sodium: 19 mg
Fiber: 1.3 g | Carbohydrates: 45.8 g | Sugar: 31.1 g

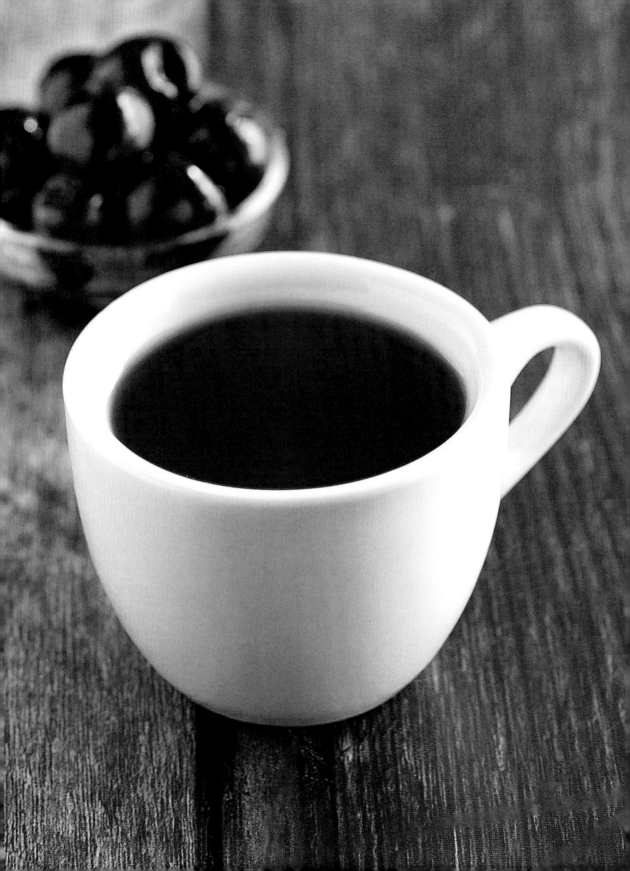

MACA HOT COCOA

Serves 2

INGREDIENTS

2 cups unsweetened vanilla almond milk
¼ cup raw cacao powder
¼ cup pure maple syrup
2 teaspoons maca root powder

---

1   In a small saucepan over low heat, gently heat the almond milk until hot.

2   Whisk in the cacao powder, maple syrup, and maca root powder until well combined and no lumps remain.

3   Serve immediately. Can be stored in an airtight container up to 1 week. May be reheated.

KEY INGREDIENT: Maca Root

Inflammation in the body can be caused by a number of different lifestyle factors. One of those is stress, especially chronic stress. Maca root is an adaptogen, which means it is a plant that naturally helps the body adapt to stressors. Adaptogens have a special ability to adapt their functions to your body's specific needs. Because of this, including maca root in your diet can help your body deal with the elements of life that cause stress, such as busy schedules, demanding work tasks, or relationship issues, thus lowering overall inflammation in the body.

This Maca Hot Cocoa is a perfect drink when stress in your life is high and you need some time to relax and rejuvenate.

Per Serving
Calories: 192 | Fat: 4.0 g | Protein: 4.0 g | Sodium: 184 mg
Fiber: 4.0 g | Carbohydrates: 38.4 g | Sugar: 25.2 g

SPICED ELDERBERRY TEA

Serves 2

INGREDIENTS

2 cups water
2 tablespoons dried elderberries
¼ teaspoon ground cinnamon
¼ teaspoon ground ginger
1 teaspoon raw honey

1 Add the water, dried elderberries, cinnamon, and ginger to a small saucepan.

2 Bring the mixture to a boil, then reduce the heat to a simmer. Allow the mixture to simmer 15 minutes.

3 Strain the elderberries using a fine-mesh strainer.

4 Stir in the honey. Serve immediately. Can be stored in an airtight container in the refrigerator up to 2 weeks. May be reheated.

KEY INGREDIENT: Elderberry

Elderberry is a plant that is commonly used medicinally throughout the world. It is well known for its ability to fight cold and flu symptoms. It is also often used as a preventative measure against falling ill, as it has been shown to stimulate the immune system.

Elderberry contains a number of different polyphenol antioxidants. One in particular, kaempferol, has potent anti-inflammatory effects. It has been shown to modulate a number of different key elements in cellular pathway links to inflammation. Kaempferol is also known to have strong anti-cancer properties, with the ability to inhibit growth of cancer cells and preserve normal cell viability.

Elderberries are also high in anthocyanins, which contribute to their anti-inflammatory properties. Anthocyanins have been shown to inhibit activation of pro-inflammatory signaling pathways in the body.

You can find dried elderberry in your local health food store, and it is widely available for purchase online.

Per Serving
Calories: 15 | Fat: 0.1 g | Protein: 0.1 g | Sodium: 0 mg
Fiber: 0.0 g | Carbohydrates: 4.1 g | Sugar: 2.9 g

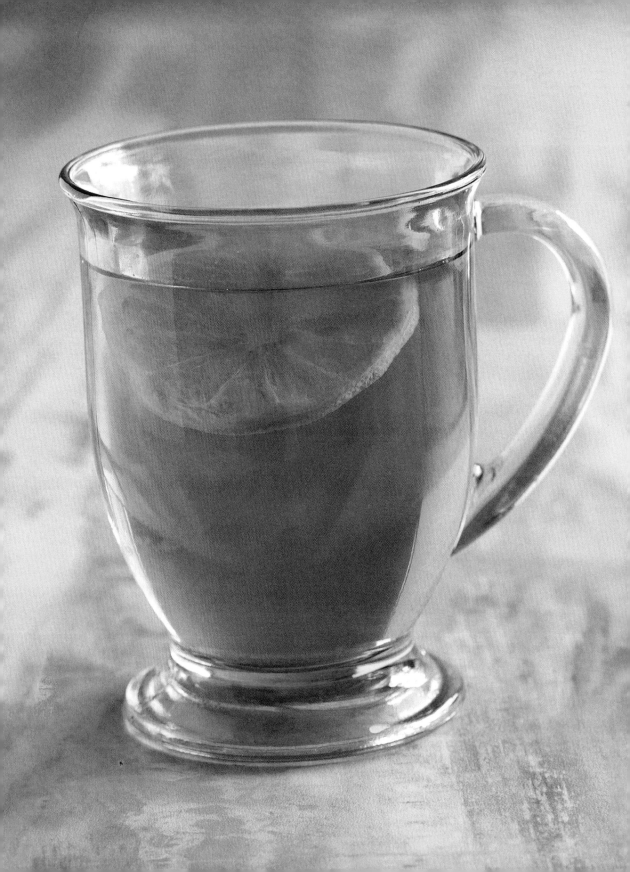

TURMERIC LEMON GREEN TEA

Serves 1

INGREDIENTS

1" piece fresh turmeric
2 tablespoons lemon juice
Pinch black pepper
1½ cups water
1 green tea bag

---

1 Peel and roughly chop the turmeric.

2 In a small saucepan, bring the turmeric, lemon juice, black pepper, and water to a simmer over low heat. Allow to simmer 3 minutes.

3 Turn off the heat, add the green tea bag, and cover the pan. Allow the tea to steep 3 minutes.

4 Remove the tea bag and strain the tea through a fine-mesh sieve.

5 Consume immediately.

KEY INGREDIENT: Lemon

Lemons are full of vitamin C, which is one of the most important antioxidants in nature. Anytime the body is exposed to free radicals, vitamin C helps neutralize them. That's one reason why vitamin C is such an important nutrient we need to make sure we're getting enough of. Vitamin C is also vital for immune system function. It's interesting to note that consuming fruits and vegetables high in vitamin C is associated with reduced risk of death from all causes. Lemons are an excellent way to help meet your vitamin C needs.

This tea recipe packs an anti-inflammatory punch with all of its ingredients and has a lovely flavor.

Per Serving
Calories: 9 | Fat: 0.1 g | Protein: 0.1 g | Sodium: 0 mg
Fiber: 0.2 g | Carbohydrates: 3.4 g | Sugar: 0.8 g

WARM WALNUT HONEY MILK

Serves 1

INGREDIENTS

⅓ cup walnut pieces
1 cup water
¼ teaspoon ground cinnamon
⅛ teaspoon pure vanilla extract
1½ teaspoons raw honey

1 Add the walnuts, water, and cinnamon to a small blender. Blend on high until the mixture is smooth.

2 Using a nut milk bag or a piece of cheesecloth, strain the milk into a small saucepan.

3 Heat the milk over medium-low heat until warm. Pour into a mug.

4 Stir in the vanilla extract and honey.

5 Serve immediately. Can be stored in an airtight container up to 1 week. May be reheated.

KEY INGREDIENT: Walnuts

Walnuts have a long, rich history, dating back to 7000 B.C. In fact, walnuts are the oldest tree food known to man. The walnut tree has always been highly revered, and its uses have included food, medicine, shelter, and dye and lamp oil.

Walnuts are a standout food because of their excellent nutritional composition. It has been found that walnuts have the highest levels of polyphenols of any nuts. Research has shown that walnuts can play a role in reducing the risk of cardiovascular disease and diabetes, both of which are related to inflammation in the body.

If you like to enjoy a warm drink before bed, this Warm Walnut Honey Milk is the perfect choice.

Per Serving
Calories: 161 | Fat: 12.9 g | Protein: 1.2 g | Sodium: 0 mg
Fiber: 0.0 g | Carbohydrates: 11.8 g | Sugar: 9.8 g

SLOW COOKER CHICKEN BONE BROTH

Serves 6

INGREDIENTS

Bones from 4 pounds chicken
8 cups cold filtered water
2 tablespoons apple cider vinegar
1 large onion, peeled and cut into chunks
2 large carrots, cut into chunks
3 stalks celery, cut into chunks
1 teaspoon sea salt
½ cup fresh parsley
3–4 sprigs fresh thyme

---

1 Put bones in a large slow cooker and cover them with water.

2 Add the rest of the ingredients to the slow cooker and allow it to sit 30–60 minutes before turning on the slow cooker.

3 Cook on low 8–24 hours. The longer time you can allow, the better.

4 Once you have finished cooking the broth, allow it to cool. Then remove the bones and vegetables from the liquid.

5 Strain broth through a fine-mesh sieve and use the back of a wooden spoon to extract all liquid from the ingredients. Repeat this procedure.

6 Store the broth in an airtight container in the refrigerator and consume within 3–5 days. May also be frozen up to 6 months.

KEY INGREDIENT: Chicken Bone Broth

Making homemade chicken bone broth is worth the time and energy it takes because the health benefits are impressive. Homemade chicken bone broth is full of minerals like calcium, phosphorus, magnesium, and potassium. Allowing the bones to sit in the liquid with apple cider vinegar before cooking is what helps draw these minerals from the bones. Bone broth also contains chondroitin sulfate and glucosamine. These are compounds that are sold as supplements to reduce inflammation, arthritis, and joint pain! Bone broth is known to heal the gut and boost the immune system, and it is great for hair, skin, and nails.

This broth is excellent for sipping on a daily basis to help reap the benefits. It can also be used for a base for your favorite soups and stews.

Per Serving
Calories: 32 | Fat: 0.3 g | Protein: 6.2 g | Sodium: 281 mg
Fiber: 0.3 g | Carbohydrates: 0.8 g | Sugar: 0.3 g

HOT SPICED APPLE ORANGE DRINK

Serves 1

INGREDIENTS

2 medium apples
1 medium orange
¼ teaspoon ground cinnamon
⅛ teaspoon ground ginger
⅛ teaspoon ground cloves

1   Prepare the apples by coring and cutting them into appropriate-sized pieces for your juicer.

2   Prepare the orange by peeling and cutting it into appropriate-sized pieces for your juicer.

3   Process the apple and orange through the juicer.

4   Strain the apple-orange juice through a fine-mesh sieve into a small saucepan.

5   Whisk the cinnamon, ginger, and cloves into the juice. Heat over medium heat until warm, about 3–4 minutes.

6   Consume immediately.

KEY INGREDIENT: Apples

"An apple a day keeps the doctor away"? Old wives' tale or truth? When you look at the nutritional information for the humble apple, it seems like a sound theory. Apples are a rich source of a number of powerful phytonutrients that can indeed keep your body healthy. All of the antioxidants in apples have been found to play an important role in cardiovascular health. The numerous antioxidants found in apples have been shown to provide protection within blood vessels. One study indicated that one apple a day for four weeks significantly reduced blood levels of oxidized LDL cholesterol. A number of the antioxidants in apples, including quercetin and catechin, have been shown to have anti-inflammatory effects.

Per Serving
Calories: 229 | Fat: 0.5 g | Protein: 1.1 g | Sodium: 3 mg
Fiber: 0.0 g | Carbohydrates: 55.7 g | Sugar: 51.7 g

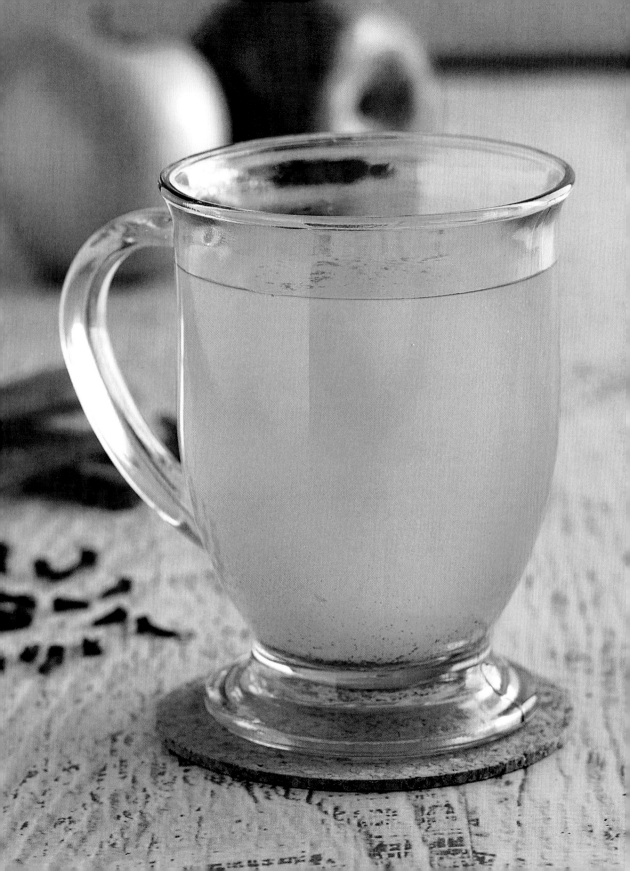

COCONUT CHAI ROOIBOS TEA LATTE

Serves 1

INGREDIENTS

1 cup water
1 red rooibos tea bag
½ cup lite canned coconut milk
1 teaspoon peeled, coarsely
    chopped fresh ginger
¼ teaspoon ground cinnamon
⅛ teaspoon ground cloves
⅛ teaspoon ground allspice
⅛ teaspoon ground cardamom
Pinch black pepper
1 teaspoon raw honey

1 In a small pan, bring the cup of water to a boil.

2 Place the tea bag in a mug and pour the boiling water over the tea bag. Allow the tea to steep 5–7 minutes.

3 While the tea is steeping, place the coconut milk, ginger, cinnamon, cloves, allspice, cardamom, and black pepper in a small blender.

4 Blend the ingredients on high until they are thoroughly combined and smooth.

5 Warm the coconut milk mixture in a small saucepan over medium heat until it is hot, about 1–2 minutes.

6 Remove the tea bag from the mug and add the coconut milk mixture.

7 Stir in the raw honey.

8 Consume immediately.

KEY INGREDIENT: Rooibos Tea

Native to South Africa, rooibos tea is an herbal remedy that's been used for centuries. The tea is extracted from the leaves of the Aspalathus linearis plant. Rooibos tea is highly regarded for its health benefits. A serving of rooibos tea provides nutrients like iron, potassium, zinc, manganese, copper, calcium, and magnesium. It's been shown to help keep hormone levels balanced, manage and prevent diabetes, help digestion issues, manage blood pressure, and prevent premature aging. Its anti-inflammatory properties result from a number of powerful compounds it contains, including quercetin.

Many of the spices in this tea recipe will also provide anti-inflammatory benefits, and it's a delicious, comforting drink.

Per Serving
Calories: 100 | Fat: 6.8 g | Protein: 0.2 g | Sodium: 9 mg
Fiber: 0.7 g | Carbohydrates: 9.3 g | Sugar: 5.9 g

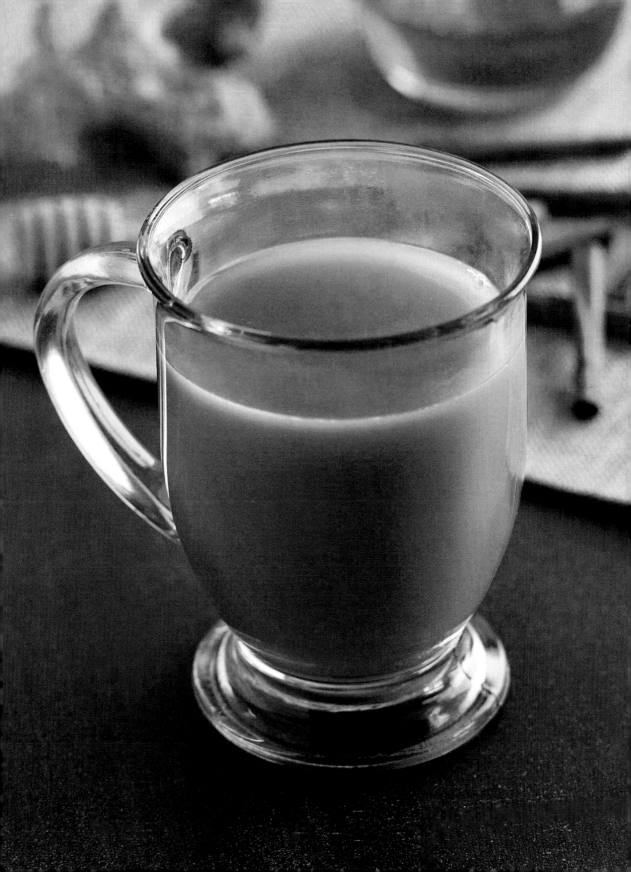

US/Metric Conversion Chart

VOLUME CONVERSIONS

US Volume Measure	Metric Equivalent
⅛ teaspoon	0.5 milliliter
¼ teaspoon	1 milliliter
½ teaspoon	2 milliliters
1 teaspoon	5 milliliters
½ tablespoon	7 milliliters
1 tablespoon (3 teaspoons)	15 milliliters
2 tablespoons (1 fluid ounce)	30 milliliters
¼ cup (4 tablespoons)	60 milliliters
⅓ cup	90 milliliters
½ cup (4 fluid ounces)	125 milliliters
⅔ cup	160 milliliters
¾ cup (6 fluid ounces)	180 milliliters
1 cup (16 tablespoons)	250 milliliters
1 pint (2 cups)	500 milliliters
1 quart (4 cups)	1 liter (about)

WEIGHT CONVERSIONS

US Weight Measure	Metric Equivalent
½ ounce	15 grams
1 ounce	30 grams
2 ounces	60 grams
3 ounces	85 grams
¼ pound (4 ounces)	115 grams
½ pound (8 ounces)	225 grams
¾ pound (12 ounces)	340 grams
1 pound (16 ounces)	454 grams

OVEN TEMPERATURE CONVERSIONS

Degrees Fahrenheit	Degrees Celsius
200 degrees F	95 degrees C
250 degrees F	120 degrees C
275 degrees F	135 degrees C
300 degrees F	150 degrees C
325 degrees F	160 degrees C
350 degrees F	180 degrees C
375 degrees F	190 degrees C
400 degrees F	205 degrees C
425 degrees F	220 degrees C
450 degrees F	230 degrees C

BAKING PAN SIZES

American	Metric
8 x 1½ inch round baking pan	20 x 4 cm cake tin
9 x 1½ inch round baking pan	23 x 3.5 cm cake tin
11 x 7 x 1½ inch baking pan	28 x 18 x 4 cm baking tin
13 x 9 x 2 inch baking pan	30 x 20 x 5 cm baking tin
2 quart rectangular baking dish	30 x 20 x 3 cm baking tin
15 x 10 x 2 inch baking pan	30 x 25 x 2 cm baking tin (Swiss roll tin)
9 inch pie plate	22 x 4 or 23 x 4 cm pie plate
7 or 8 inch springform pan	18 or 20 cm springform or loose bottom cake tin
9 x 5 x 3 inch loaf pan	23 x 13 x 7 cm or 2 lb narrow loaf or pate tin
1½ quart casserole	1.5 liter casserole
2 quart casserole	2 liter casserole

Index

To Your Health!

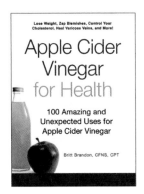

Lose Weight, Zap Blemishes, Control Your
Cholesterol, Heal Varicose Veins, and More!

Apple Cider Vinegar
for Health

100 Amazing and
Unexpected Uses for
Apple Cider Vinegar

Britt Brandon, CFNS, CPT

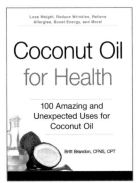

Lose Weight, Reduce Wrinkles, Relieve
Allergies, Boost Energy, and More!

Coconut Oil
for Health

100 Amazing and
Unexpected Uses for
Coconut Oil

Britt Brandon, CFNS, CPT

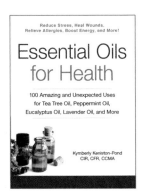

Reduce Stress, Heal Wounds,
Relieve Allergies, Boost Energy, and More!

Essential Oils
for Health

100 Amazing and Unexpected Uses
for Tea Tree Oil, Peppermint Oil,
Eucalyptus Oil, Lavender Oil, and More

Kymberly Keniston-Pond
CIR, CFR, CCMA

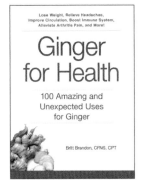

Lose Weight, Relieve Headaches,
Improve Circulation, Boost Immune System,
Alleviate Arthritis Pain, and More!

Ginger
for Health

100 Amazing and
Unexpected Uses
for Ginger

Britt Brandon, CFNS, CPT

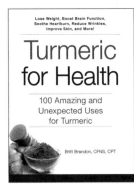

Lose Weight, Boost Brain Function,
Soothe Heartburn, Reduce Wrinkles,
Improve Skin, and More!

Turmeric
for Health

100 Amazing and
Unexpected Uses
for Turmeric

Britt Brandon, CFNS, CPT

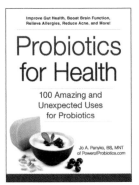

Improve Gut Health, Boost Brain Function,
Relieve Allergies, Reduce Acne, and More!

Probiotics
for Health

100 Amazing and
Unexpected Uses
for Probiotics

Jo A. Panyko, BS, MNT
of PowerofProbiotics.com

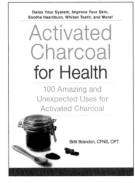

Detox Your System, Improve Your Skin,
Soothe Heartburn, Whiten Teeth, and More!

Activated Charcoal
for Health

100 Amazing and
Unexpected Uses for
Activated Charcoal

Britt Brandon, CFNS, CPT

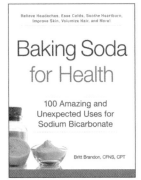

Relieve Headaches, Ease Colds, Soothe Heartburn,
Improve Skin, Volumize Hair, and More!

Baking Soda
for Health

100 Amazing and
Unexpected Uses for
Sodium Bicarbonate

Britt Brandon, CFNS, CPT

PICK UP OR DOWNLOAD YOUR COPIES TODAY!

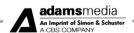

adamsmedia
An Imprint of Simon & Schuster
A CBS COMPANY